Motivational Strategies
in
Geriatric
Rehabilitation

Mark S. Rosenfeld, PhD, OTR/L
Editor

The American Occupational Therapy Association, Inc.

Disclaimers

"This publication is designed to provide accurate and authoritative information in regard to the subject matter covered. It is sold or distributed with the understanding that the publisher is not engaged in rendering legal, accounting, or other professional service. If legal advice or other expert assistance is required, the services of a competent professional person should be sought."

> —From the Declaration of Principles jointly adopted by the
> American Bar Association and a Committee of Publishers and Associations

It is the objective of the American Occupational Therapy Association to be a forum for free expression and interchange of ideas. The opinions expressed by the contributors to this work are their own and not necessarily those of either the editors or the American Occupational Therapy Association.

ISBN 1-56900-060-3

Designer: Carolyn Uhl
Photographer: Donna McIvor Joss
Printed in the United States of America

Acknowledgments

The following listing is meant to recognize the contributions of individuals and groups whose efforts have made this book a reality. The text is dedicated to Arthur and Lillian Rosenfeld, who raised me and recently taught me a great deal about living well as elders.

Mark S. Rosenfeld, PhD, OTR/L, Editor

Assistant Professor, Worcester State College, Worcester MA

Geriatric Practice, TheraTx, Inc.

Certified Psychotherapist

Consultant, *Improving Treatment Compliance in Geriatric Rehabilitation*

Thanks are extended to TheraTx, Inc., for assistance in generating case study vignettes for this book.

CHAPTER AUTHORS

Warren F. Dahlin, Jr., MS, OTR/L
Assistant Professor of Health Care Administration, Director of Gerontology Program, Stonehill College, North Easton MA

Susan Fasoli, MS, OTR/L
Instructor, Worcester State College, Worcester MA

Geriatric Practice, Walpole Area Visiting Nurses Association, Walpole MA

Rick Fentin, MED, CFP
Certified Financial Planner and Rehabilitation Counselor

Investment Advisory Association, The Acacia Group, Waltham MA

Paul J. Goldberg, MSW, LICSW
Social Work Supervisor, Visiting Nurses Association, Cambridge MA

Janice Hengel, MGA, MS, OTR/L
Psychogeriatric Practice, Newtown PA

Karen McCarthy, COTA/L
Geriatric Practice, Team Rehabilitation, Inc., Worcester MA

Virginia J. Morgan, OTR/L
Director of Occupational Therapy,
Spaulding Rehabilitation Hospital,
Boston MA

Vickie Patterson, OTR
Occupational Therapy Clinical
Manager, Visiting Nurse Association of
Texas, Dallas TX

Paul N. Petrone, MOT/L
Occupational Therapy Supervisor,
Spaulding Rehabilitation Hospital,
Boston MA

Martin Proulx, COTA/L
Geriatric Practice, Team Rehabilitation,
Worcester MA

Robert R. Read, EdD
Psychologist, Harvard University,
Bureau of Study Counsel
Faculty, Cambridge College

Psychologist, Private Practice,
Belmont MA

Kim Watkins, BS, OTR/L
Occupational Therapy Supervisor,
Charles V. Hogan Regional Center,
Danvers MA

John D. Weagraff, Jr., PSYD, PhD
Director of Pastoral Services,
Westborough State Hospital,
Westborough MA

Staff Psychologist, Community
Counseling Center of Blackstone
Valley, Inc.

Susan K. Weiner, OTR/L, MPH
Director of Occupational Therapy,
Charles V. Hogan Regional Center,
Danvers MA

PHOTOGRAPHER

Donna McIvor Joss, EDD, OTR/L
Chair, Occupational Therapy
Department, Worcester State College,
Worcester MA

**CASE STUDY ANALYSIS
EXPERTS**

**Jacqueline R. Brennan, MS, OTR/L,
RPT/L**
Assistant Professor, Worcester State
College, Worcester MA

Susan Fasoli, MS, OTR/L
Instructor, Worcester State College,
Worcester MA

Geriatric Practice, Walpole Area
Visiting Nurses Association,
Walpole MA

Gail S. Fidler, OTR, FAOTA
Scholar in Residence, College of
Misericordia, Division of Allied Health
Professions, Dallas PA

Joanne M. Gallagher, MS, OTR/L
Instructor, Worcester State College,
Worcester MA

Cynthia Kennealy, COTA/L, OTS
Geriatric Practice, TheraTx, Inc.,
Worcester, MA

Cheryl Lucas, MS, OTR/L
Licensed Nursing Home Administrator,
Homecare Therapist, MA

**Michael Pizzi, MS, OTR/L, CHES,
FAOTA**
Founder, Positive Images and Wellness,
Inc., Silver Spring MD

Mark S. Rosenfeld, PhD, OTR/L
Assistant Professor, Worcester State College, Worcester MA
Geriatric Practice, TheraTx, Inc.
Certified Psychotherapist
Consultant, Improving Treatment Compliance in Geriatric Rehabilitation

Jane Sorensen, PhD, OTR/L
Private Practice, New York NY
Columnist, OT Advance

Janet H. Watts, MS, OTR/C
Associate Professor, Virginia Commonwealth University, Medical College of Virginia, Richmond VA

Gail Wolfe, MBA, OTR/L
Rehabilitation Program Manager, TheraTx, Inc., Worcester, MA

CASE STUDY VIGNETTE CONTRIBUTORS

Rhoda Dorfzaun, OTR/L
Mount Lebanon Manor, Pittsburgh PA

Susan Fasoli, MS, OTR/L
Instructor, Worcester State College, Worcester MA
Geriatric Practice, Walpole Area Visiting Nurses Association, Walpole MA

Kelley Drane Fleming, OTR/L
Spaulding Rehabilitation Hospital, Boston MA

Maura Hinkle, OTR/L
Director of Occupational Therapy, Mount Lebanon Manor, Pittsburgh PA

Marianne Fung, OTR/L
TheraTx, Inc., Worcester, MA

Joanne Gallagher, MS, OTR/L
Instructor, Worcester State College, Worcester MA

Ute Gruner, OTR/L
TheraTx, Inc., Worcester, MA

Karen Halfon, OTR/L
Spaulding Rehabilitation Hospital, Boston MA

Marcy Lee, OTR/L
Emerson Hospital, Concord MA

Cheryl Lucas, MS, OTR/L
Licensed Nursing Home Administrator, Homecare Therapist, MA

Renee Lundfelt, OTR/L
TheraTx, Inc., Worcester, MA

Dawn Morrill, MS, OTR
Visiting Nurses Association of Texas, Dallas TX

Patty Pierce, OTS
Worcester State College, Worcester MA

Susan Pierce, COTA/L
Mount Lebanon Manor, Pittsburgh PA

Virginia Smith, OTR/L
Emerson Hospital, Concord MA

Jane Sorensen, PhD, OTR/L
Private Practice, New York NY
Columnist, OT Advance

Janice Walker, OTR
Visiting Nurses Association of Texas, Dallas TX

Preface

After many years of occupational therapy practice in mental health, I began part-time work in geriatric rehabilitation in addition to teaching at Worcester State College. Physical disabilities was a new focus for me, and so I entered the culture of nursing homes and subacute rehabilitation with an outsider's perspective. On the other hand, I certainly possessed an insider's view of my profession.

I learned a great deal in 3 years. My technical skills improved. I came to respect the knowledge, commitment, and efficiency of the therapists I encountered. However, I also observed many forces that limited occupational therapy practice to a narrow domain, which discouraged a holistic understanding of patients and the use of a full range of occupations in treatment. I often encountered therapists who met the daily requirements for reimbursable "mods" of treatment but who were dissatisfied with their jobs. Some hopped from one rehabilitation company to another, searching for something better.

When practice moves so quickly that the identity, life history, occupational preferences, and motivations of the individual cannot be addressed, then treatment becomes a rote, technical procedure for therapist and patient alike. When the culture of supervision is weak as well, therapists have little opportunity to reflect on their successes and failures. Professional growth falters.

In subacute practice, while therapists often could not embrace the "whole lives" of their patients, the patients often felt that their whole lives were on the line. A fractured hip, a stroke, an amputation, a heart attack, or sudden worsening of diseases are traumatic occurences in the lives of older people. They worry they will die or never return home to restore the life context they value. They are among strangers who do not know their life accomplishments, family members, or significant losses. In addition, pain, depression, anxiety, and cognitive deficits compromise treatment motivation for many of these patients, yet real rehabilitation requires the patient's motivation to act.

In such a context, subacute occupational therapy treatment must be seen as a form of crisis intervention. Functional improvement is a meaningful element of intervention if it truly helps to restore life context, hope, and purpose in existence. Evaluating functional skills with numerical ratings on a scale can be systematic and efficient. If it occurs in a practice environment that values only such ratings, however, then the complexity of human functioning is trivialized and deconstructed—and so is our professional practice.

Given my concern for a holistic approach to treatment and my expertise in mental health, I began to search in clinical experience and in professional literature for an integrated approach. I believe that I and the many others who have contributed to this book have found theories and methods that support a holistic integration of motivation and action in geriatric physical rehabilitation. Implementing this approach has in no way reduced my efficiency in producing reimbursable treatment "mods." My hope is that this book will be a resource and a stimulus, one that will help us keep our eyes on the prize—effective, holistic, collaborative, and occupationally based practice.

Table of Contents

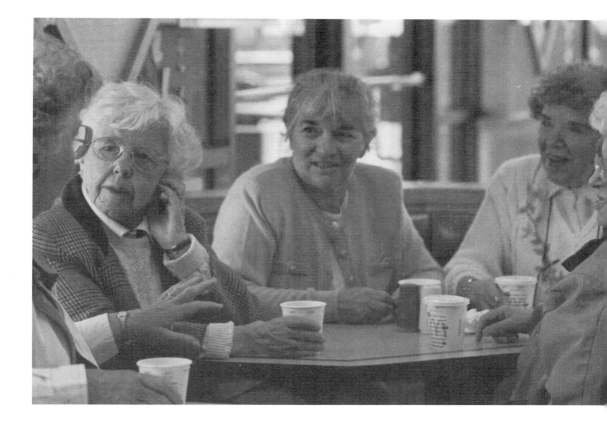

Introduction

This book has several goals. The first is to provide a theoretical and practical way to approach coping and adaptation from an occupational perspective. Many excellent resources already support therapists' thinking about biomedical issues. A second goal is to describe the application of a motivational approach to patient assessment, to current documentation and reimbursement systems, and to the development of a group program. Finally, the third, and perhaps most important, goal is to create an interactive resource of case problems and recommendations for classroom study and for clinical problem solving.

The use of "paper" cases and role-played clinical interactions has received considerable attention as elements of a problem-based learning approach (Van Leit, 1995). By studying realistic clinical problems, learners strengthen the procedural, interactive, and conditional reasoning required in practice. According to Fleming (1991), procedural reasoning enables the therapist to select and apply appropriate treatment techniques. Through interactive reasoning, the therapist accesses and understands the patient's perspective about occupation, illness, treatment, and recovery. Conditional reasoning also helps to design and refine a coherent view of the patient's future functioning and life options.

Therapists cannot speak directly with the experts who have written case recommendations for this book. Reading case problems and solutions is not a substitute for face-to-face supervision. It is, however, a kind of supervision, since it uses theory to enlighten clinical situations, suggests specific action plans, and encourages the reader toward creative clinical reasoning.

While such reading may validate or challenge one's thinking, it is clear that a therapist must develop his or her own effective style of interacting with patients and resolving treatment problems. Therefore, the studies are offered as relevant examples rather than as prescriptive recipes for treatment. Nonetheless, the studies include real clinical dilemmas experienced by geriatric occupational therapists across the country and "supervisory" responses by some of the brightest and most experienced clinicians and theorists in our profession.

SUGGESTIONS FOR USING THIS BOOK: FOR SUPERVISORS, THERAPISTS, INSTRUCTORS, STUDENTS, OTRS, AND COTAS

The intention of the editors, authors, and publisher is that this book be an accessible and practical resource. We hope each copy will become dog-eared and worn with use by many therapists, educators, and students. The organization, contents, and writing style are designed for busy people who need immediate information that can be translated quickly into clinical action. It has been a challenge to produce a book that addresses the needs of occupational therapy students, educators, COTAs, and OTRs. The following are suggestions for effective use of the book.

Chapter 1 frames the issues of aging, disability, and rehabilitation. Reading chapter 2 is essential. The case vignettes and responses are based upon the philosophy, system analysis, and theories explained in this section. Critical treatment planning and program development concepts are introduced as well.

Therapists in need of practical ideas for treatment may locate relevant examples among the case studies in chapter 3. The cases were submitted by participating therapists from acute, subacute, long-term-care, and home-care practice settings. Amputations, fractures, cerebrovascular accidents (CVAs), coronary artery bypass graft, osteoarthritis, joint replacement, postpolio syndrome, alcohol dependence, bereavement, mental

retardation, and impending death are among the medical problems represented. Cases are titled according to the motivational dilemma they present. An expert has responded to each case. In a few instances, the same therapist wrote a case description and discussed the treatment strategies he or she used.

The introductory case in chapter 3 provides a terrific illustration of the complex issues and decisions intrinsic to geriatric occupational therapy practice. Students may read and discuss this case for its consciousness-building value. The author for this section also has presented some important suggestions for understanding the interplay of cognitive deficits and reduced motivation.

Educators may assign students a specific case for classroom treatment planning or for homework. Students should cover the expert's response while reading and considering the case material. Students then can write their own explanations of the nuclear problem, formulate a goal for motivational intervention, describe intervention strategies, and specify the nuclear tasks for problem resolution and restoration of life context. Having completed these steps individually or in a group, students may wish to read the case response written by the expert.

It is important to recognize that understandings, ideas, and plans that differ from those of the experts are not inherently wrong. Varied approaches may be effective in addressing the same treatment problem. Each therapist develops a unique clinical style and techniques. Nonetheless, the experts' recommendations illustrate the application of concepts to realistic practice situations and will help to refine and deepen the clinical reasoning skills of the reader. Rehabilitation managers may use a similar method for inservice training to strengthen therapists' motivational intervention skills.

Chapter 4 offers practical advice for effective documentation and reimbursement of motivational interventions. In the current health care environment, this is an indispensable component for implementation of the approach advocated in this book.

Chapters 5, 6, and 7 offer perspectives about occupational therapy treatment with special populations of psychogeriatric and developmentally disabled patients and under unique conditions of home and community-based practice.

Chapters 8 and 9 provide valuable ideas about the benefits and design of successful group programs in acute and subacute treatment settings.

The influences of finances and religion on treatment motivation are discussed in chapters 10 and 11. A holistic approach requires consideration of many dimensions in the patient's life. While exploration of family and culture are not addressed in separate sections, case vignettes and responses offer appropriate attention to these factors.

Finally, a systematic approach to evaluating motivation and rehabilitation potential is proposed in chapter 12. Clearly, a great deal of work remains before occupational therapists can bolster our clinical judgments in this area with valid assessment tools.

Any and all uses of this book are intended to stimulate reflection on the quality of clinical practice. I genuinely hope that the book will assist therapists in advocating for and designing holistic interventions and in reclaiming a broad domain of concern for occupational therapy practice in geriatric rehabilitation.

REFERENCES

Fleming, M. (1991). The therapist with the three-track mind. *American Journal of Occupational Therapy, 45*, 1007–1014.

Van Leit, B. (1995). Using the case method to develop clinical reasoning skills in problem-based learning. *American Journal of Occupational Therapy, 49*, 349–353.

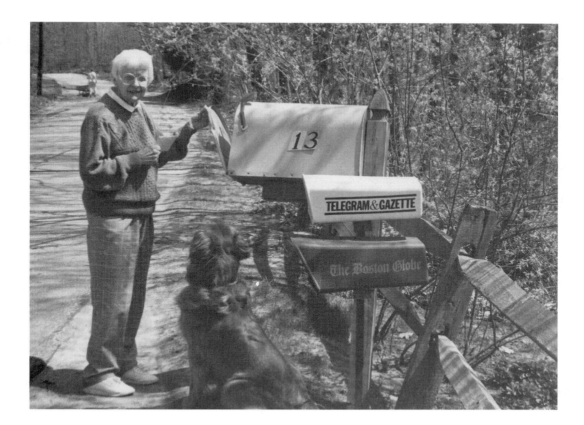

Chapter **1** *Ambivalence about Aging and Health Care in America*

Mark S. Rosenfeld, PhD, OTR/L

We are all getting older. Because of demographic shifts and advances in medicine, the proportion of Americans over age 65 continues to grow. By the year 2025, it is estimated that one-fifth of our population will be in this category (Cohen, 1993). Longer life is not simply a trend of the 1990s. The human life span has doubled over the last 3 million years. We now live twice as long as the next longest-lived primates (Pearson & Shaw, 1982).

The increase in numbers of older people has brought issues, conflicts, and innovations related to aging into intense public awareness. Longevity, it seems, can be perceived as a blessing or a curse, depending on the health, relationships, and financial standing of the individual. While medical systems take heroic measures to preserve the lives of gravely ill older people, living wills and "Do Not Resuscitate" orders are written to allow the end of lives overcome by pain or devoid of meaning.

Society is ambivalent about older people for other reasons as well. While many are pleased to have parents and grandparents who live longer, ageism creates negative perceptions of older people. Many ignore the continued contributions of elders and forget that their past accomplishments made our present comforts possible (Beers & Urice, 1992).

Many Americans are concerned about the costly health care and entitlement resources older people claim. Elders already account for almost half of all days of hospital care in the United States (American Association of Retired Persons & Administration on Aging, 1990). Nearly half our health care dollars are expended treating patients in their last year of life (Collen, 1993).

While many argue for the moral obligation to provide such care, many others argue strongly against its practical value (Felts, 1993).

Conflicts about services for elders are reflected in government policies and initiatives. The White House Conference on Aging (1995) set as its ideal, "Generations Aging Together with Independence, Opportunity, and Dignity." The conference endorsed proposals to continue and strengthen Medicare and Social Security programs. At the same time, Congress considered cuts and massive restructuring of the Medicare Program, limiting physician, patient, and family health care choices (Christenson, 1995).

LIFESTYLE EVOLUTION AND INNOVATION

The lifestyles of older Americans are changing. In many instances, the rocking chair stands idle while its supposed occupant is on the move. Elder services' vans pick up many people daily to promote and preserve their community involvement. Many seniors continue to drive. Now they can participate in elder driver safety classes for at least 8 hours a year to maintain their skills and also qualify for a reduction in auto insurance.

The average retirement for American workers spans about 20 years. The financial requirements over such a long period bring many people out of retirement and encourage others to retain their careers far beyond age 65. While work may be a boon to more healthy elders, it is a burden to others. Some younger people also perceive that desired positions in the workforce are unavailable, occupied by elders reluctant to retire.

Older travelers have breathed new life into the tourism industry. Groups of elders are frequent visitors to Alaska, Europe, the Far East, and even Antarctica. Recreational vehicles driven by retirees wander the countryside. Elder-hostel programs draw seniors to universities around the country to study and discuss an amazing range of subjects.

Today's elders are beginning to take control of lifestyle factors that affect their health. Many thousands have quit smoking. Adherence to low-fat and low-sodium diets is common. Aerobic exercise regimens and strength training is pursued by many as well. Vitamins and dietary supplements are taken in daily rituals along with medications. Elders in sunny climates are often careful in using sunscreen and clothing to protect their skin. Many individuals have become savvy consumers of the latest information about health and prevention of disease.

Evolving innovations have increased and improved living environment options for older adults. Retirement communities and condominiums abound. Home-care services, assisted living, congregate living, and subacute nursing home beds are part of a new and flexible continuum of settings congruent with changing health care needs of individuals. While these options represent progress, it is possible that they may contribute unwittingly to segmentation and isolation of some elders from family members and from contact with people of diverse ages and experiences.

SICKNESS AND HEALTH: A DEVELOPMENTAL CHALLENGE

Aging as a process presents some unique contradictions and challenges. While physical and mental deterioration seem inexorable for some, improved health, deepening knowledge, and wisdom accrue to others. Long experience and relationships can create clarity about one's capacities and priorities. Such strengths help people to enjoy themselves and to cope with the problems of aging. While mortality is a fact of human life, advanced age is a dynamic state that can be strongly influenced by activity, attitude, exercise, and nutrition (Evans & Rosenberg, 1991). As a result, maintaining the quality of life is a personal developmental challenge for every older person.

An older woman once spent a half hour describing her numerous medical problems. Finally, she paused, chuckled, and apologized for giving an "organ recital." The majority of older people could give such a recital. As people age, destructive forces are at work. Tissues, cells, and molecules deteriorate. The repair/destruction ratio declines as older adults are less able to repair the damage of the years. Accumulated damage tends to promote more damage (Pearson & Shaw, 1982). As compared with younger counterparts, elders have more diseases. Their illnesses often involve a combination of abnormalities, organ systems, and body parts. Therefore, they require more diagnostic and therapeutic procedures. They use more office visits, see more medical specialists, spend more days in hospitals, and take more medications. Older people recuperate more slowly. They are more vulnerable to stress and have weakened immune responses (Collen, 1993). The most common medical conditions affecting elders include hypertension, diabetes, heart disease, and osteoarthritis. All these ailments require continuing, rather than episodic, medical care (Felts, 1993). An ironic joke from a state with a large senior citizen concentration quips that the sound of ambulance sirens is the music of Florida. It is no wonder that

the health care of older Americans costs a great deal.

Apart from the disease process, a portion of the disabling changes attributed to aging are caused by *sarcopenia*, the combined affects of immobility, lack of exertion, and dependency (Evans & Rosenberg, 1991). These factors cause insidious weakening of body structures, decreased muscle mass, increased fat content, and gradual weakening of functional capacities. In some instances, depression associated with loss, illness, and old age may contribute to development of a sedentary lifestyle (Coleman, 1984). In several studies, 15 to 30 percent of older people have been found to have depressive symptoms, and the percentage is significantly higher for those with dementia (Lazarus, Newton, Cohle, et al., 1987).

Billig (1993) suggests that there are "three ways to approach one's aging: bemoan its arrival and pay a great deal of attention to every change that aging brings; accept the notion passively that getting older is better than the alternative and do the best one can; and try actively to overcome the facts that the body is deteriorating and the mind is not as fast as it used to be and try to do as many of the things one wants to do" (p. xi). While the last approach is considered preferable, people generally draw from each approach at various times and in varying amounts.

MODELS OF SERVICE: A CRITICAL ISSUE

The roles of occupational therapists and the services we provide, document, and for which we are reimbursed, define our profession. Current practice is shaped by countervailing forces that confuse rather than solidify professional identity. These forces include product-oriented reimbursement standards; a profit-driven health system; occupational therapy literature favoring collaborative, holistic models for evaluation and treatment; and a powerful but uncertain health reform initiative in Washington. While AOTA's political action committee asks our support for lobbying to protect and promote occupational therapy, other voices urge us to exert moral and ethical leadership, and to act in the public interest and not merely out of self-interest (AOTA, 1995; Yerxa & Sharrott, 1986).

A holistic approach to understanding motivation for treatment and strategic use of occupation are advocated in this book. It is important to explain and justify these positions, but it is crucial to recognize the constraints therapists face in implementing such methods, and to identify practical ways to overcome them.

THE ARGUMENT FOR HOLISM IN GERIATRIC REHABILITATION

Levine and Gitlin (1993) observe that occupational therapy services and treatment approaches are primarily based on an acute care medical model. This model emphasizes a symptom-based, time-limited approach and therapist-driven strategies to promote functional independence, often through increases in subcomponent skills. As previously described, the needs of elderly patients with multiple, chronic conditions require continuity of care. Cost containment efforts of managed care companies, in contrast, dictate narrow windows of treatment opportunity. Severely limited time frames for therapy and a high rate of job mobility among therapists create a fragmented context for treatment. The needs of elderly patients are frequently not well served by the current model.

Complex life changes accompany such chronic, disabling conditions. Therefore, the goals and issues of patients and caregivers related to daily activities must be incorporated into treatment that encompasses a holistic perspective of the patient's life (Bonder, 1994; Clark, Corcoran, & Gitlin, 1995). While reimbursement standards often require quantifiable improvements, Ory and Williams (1989) find that goals stated by older adult patients often seem qualitative. These researchers believe that addressing patients' goals incrementally is most effective. Through small, meaningful successes in occupations relevant to the individual, a cognitive bridge is built between former occupations and new physical and emotional needs.

To identify occupations that mobilize the will and effort of an individual, therapists must understand that person's life story. "The volitional process involves the telling and living of a personal narrative situated in a cultural and historical context" (Helfrich, Kielhofner & Mattingly, 1994, p. 316). Therapeutic relationships that enable such telling and understanding require that therapists be *covenantors* (collaborators and friends), in addition to good technicians or parental advisors (Peloquin, 1990).

Bonder (1993) and Pelland (1987) argue that effective functional assessment must address motivation, meaning, and life satisfaction issues. Only then can therapists determine the personal and environmental forces that prevent or foster performance.

Health professionals and consumers are worried that health care reform will seriously curtail the provision of services. There are strong indications, however, that the upcoming changes will focus strongly on functional improvement as well as cost containment. Our ability to measure functional, occupational changes will then be more important than documentation regarding subcomponent skills (Berthelette & Lewis, 1995).

If this analysis is accurate, then a great opportunity for occupational therapy will emerge. Service models can then be promoted that include motivational assessment and intervention and address work and leisure roles as well as self-care and activities of daily living (ADL) skills (Friedland & Renwick, 1993). In such a context, the quality of life would achieve equal status with the quantity of performances. Reflecting and planning would be reimbursed along with doing. And occupation might become therapists' preferred method for subcomponent skill development.

To create such an outcome, occupational therapists must concentrate on their ability to understand and measure function. We must articulate and systematically assess the connections between motivation and performance. A cause-and-effect relationship between occupational therapy treatment and functional improvement has been supported by meta-analysis of 15 studies (Carlson, Fanchiang, Zemke, & Clark, 1996). The case for these benefits can only be firmly established through continued research. Legislators, third-party payers, and the public must be convinced of the critical value of occupation to human life. Stronger ties with consumer advocacy groups would add strength and credibility to our arguments and make us more than another special interest looking for a larger piece of the health care pie.

CONSTRAINTS INHIBITING HOLISTIC OCCUPATIONAL THERAPY PRACTICE

Despite the opportunities that health care reform may hold, powerful forces have driven geriatric occupational therapy practice into a narrow and pressured context. These forces have pushed practice toward reductionistic evaluation and treatment methods. Many therapists have become preoccupied with subcomponent skill development, while deemphasizing reflective, collaborative relationships with patients. The therapist in the trenches is familiar with these trends and is frequently frustrated by them. The description that follows presents a worst-case perspective in order to highlight some of the influences limiting occupational therapy practice. Some practical suggestions are offered.

Time

Geriatric occupational therapists move through the work day at the speed of light. A number of factors account for this extreme pace. Patients have limited coverage for treatment days and limitations on the length of each session because of cost-containment efforts. Progress must occur quickly to justify continued care. Therapists' billing is determined by documented units of service. Therefore, corporate goals to maximize profits press therapists to produce as many billable units as possible per day.

These time pressures discourage therapists from reflecting and planning with patients and from learning about their lives in detail. They inhibit the use of personally relevant occupations in favor of standard procedures, exercises, and equipment that may be quickly used with a broad spectrum of patients. Finally, they influence therapists to see patient motivation as an internal trait. If that commodity is lacking, the therapist is often too busy to examine the interactional process components that are interfering.

Goals

In the time- and outcome-pressured context described above, evaluation is often quick, routinized, and performed "on" more than "with" the patient. The evaluation provides a fragmented mobility, ADL, and cognitive snapshot of the patient at a moment in time. Beyond medical data and previous living situation, the chart contains little information about the patient's life. Some evidence of previous ADL performance is necessary to demonstrate a functional slide and to determine rehabilitation potential. If the patient was more functionally independent in the recent past, it is thought that he or she may be able to regain premorbid skills.

Ill, injured, or postoperative and new to the setting, the patient may not immediately be able to formulate cogent and realistic goals. He or she may not have a clear concept of the medical prognosis or the rehabilitation process. Frequently, the therapist elicits some basic statements from the patient about desires for the future. The therapist then uses the functional snapshot data to predict and quantify rehabilitation outcomes in each of the areas stipulated on a reimbursement-driven form.

This goal-setting procedure favors standard outcome expectations while deemphasizing individual preferences, histories, and motivations. Treatment goals address subcomponent skills, self-care, ADL, and mobility skills, which lend themselves to easy measurement. This measurement is critical, since comparative outcome measures will be used to document and justify future treatment. Leisure, work, and social goals are frequently unrepresented in the evaluation or treatment plan. It is assumed that these areas are not supported by Medicare and other reimbursers. Therefore, they become irrelevant to patient treatment and are eliminated from the occupational therapy domain of concern.

Role Definitions

In the current environment, competing and complementary roles seem to limit an appropriately broad role definition for occupational therapy. Activity personnel, not occupational therapists, have become the purveyors of occupation in many clinical settings. Unfortunately, these small activity departments are only able to meet diversional and mental health needs for many patients through group activities and outings. Activity personnel are not trained nor logistically able to assess and provide individualized occupational interventions. While some therapists manage to incorporate occupations beyond ADL practice into their treatment methods, they often do so without the support of institutional culture.

Psychosocial problems frequently affect the rehabilitation process (Versluys, 1995). Occupational therapists may recognize depression, anger, anxiety, psychosis, adjustment disorders, and learned helplessness in their patients. However, therapists do not often see their professional role or skills as encompassing treatment of these problems. They may be instrumental in generating a psychiatric consultation for a troubled patient, but do not systematically plan and implement intervention strategies to address psychosocial issues. Although occupational therapy universally includes course work and fieldwork related to physical dysfunction and psychosocial dysfunction, the latter skills have not been maintained in nonholistic treatment venues. Therapists also expect that reimbursement for motivational and psychosocial interventions will be resisted by third party payers. Kern (1994) has indicated that this assumption is generally incorrect.

Great teamwork often occurs among occupational, physical, and speech therapists to the benefit of patients. These professions as well as nursing staff occupy patient care roles that overlap with occupational therapy. Rather than attempt a detailed analysis of areas of overlap, I ask the reader to recognize that our role in geriatric rehabilitation is defined in a populated environment. We make room for others. We concede areas of special knowledge and expertise. They, in turn, expect certain functions of us in designing therapeutic programs. This shared responsibility breeds comfort and complacency and/or conflict and competition. Whichever climate predominates, each profession is not only enhanced but also clearly limited by the presence of the others. It is an interesting exercise to ask oneself, "How would I define geriatric occupational therapy practice without the need to consider the juxtaposition of other disciplines?"

Space and Supplies

Space allocations vary considerably. Some settings provide separate occupational therapy areas or rooms. Others combine rehabilitation services in a large multiple-use environment. Space and supplies symbolize the relative importance of services and treatment methods.

Equipment frequently observed in these settings includes walkers and mats for mobility training, standing tables, exercise pulleys, hot and cold packs, and ergometers. An ADL closet or cabinet contains adaptive equipment for feeding, bathing, dressing, and grooming assistance. Pegboards, stacking cones, and clothespin boxes are present as well, along with splinting materials. The only occupational resource regularly present is a kitchen area with appliances, utensils, and supplies for kitchen evaluation and practice. Without a broader range of occupational supplies, therapists dealing with physical dysfunction cannot easily address a full spectrum of community living skills (Neistadt & Seymour, 1995; Taylor & Manguno, 1991).

A creative subacute rehabilitation manager with whom I worked bought flower bulbs for a patient to plant one spring. She arranged for another patient to use a computer from the business office. We conspired to borrow knitting supplies, playing cards, and water colors from the activities department. We also found some collating work in the rehabilitation office for a cognitively disabled former clerical worker. I have often requested the activities staff to specifically include a patient in a relevant activity program for therapeutic reasons.

As a result of strong disincentives in many acute and subacute physical disabilities settings, the broad application of occupation seems to press beyond the usual scope of practice. Occupational interventions are not often documented, despite their targeted therapeutic value. The necessary supplies are not stocked and are not provided for in the occupational therapy budget. If they were, I believe therapists would use varied occupations in a timely and effective way. To do so, however, many therapists would need some reorientation. Some have forgotten the value of occupation after leaving school and learning the ways of the clinic. Others attended occupational therapy programs that abandoned the teaching of varied occupations because society and health systems devalued them while elevating the importance of technologies over the past 20 years.

Is the occupational pendulum swinging back? Will work, leisure, chores, and rest become the basis for occupational therapy practice once again? This is unclear. As previously stated, there are pendular forces in occupational therapy in health care and in society, swinging in both directions— toward holism and occupation, and toward reductionism and isolated subcomponent skills.

The Profit Motive

Health care is truly a big business, with 1995 revenues in excess of $1 trillion. Geriatric health is a strong and rapidly growing area. Profitability has increased the demand for occupational therapy personnel and driven up salaries for geriatric specialists, although these trends may already be shifting. Occupational therapy revenues, in fact, have been the engine for profits in this area, since physical therapy reimbursement is capitated and speech therapy referrals are much less numerous.

Acute hospital and rehabilitation hospital profits depend on consistent performance under pressure. Length of stay in these settings is short (1–7 days) and increasingly controlled by managed care. As patients are discharged, hospitals must fill now-empty beds or suffer losses. Marketing services to physicians and health maintenance organizations

(HMOs) has become a central activity in successful companies and institutions. To attract referrals, rehabilitation teams must build a record of successful treatment within managed care utilization parameters.

These pressures are felt in the competitive subacute and home-care markets as well. Profits in Medicaid supporting long-term care are obviously not connected as tightly to treatment outcomes or length of stay. In subacute settings, profits often are shared by nursing homes and rehabilitation contractors. This arrangement contributes to a volatile and highly mobile climate in which therapists frequently change jobs for better salaries, benefits, or working conditions. Nursing homes often terminate contracts with rehabilitation companies, seeking a better arrangement with that company's competitors. In order to eliminate the need to split profits, some nursing homes are attempting to hire their own rehabilitation teams. Nationwide rehabilitation companies, meanwhile, are merging with and buying nursing home chains to strengthen their positions in an uncertain business.

Should Congress capitate occupational therapy or significantly limit services to consumers, the current system of geriatric rehabilitation could come apart at the seams. The next incarnation is anybody's guess. No doubt, the reader has seen beyond the author's current knowledge as new legislation and system adaptations have unfolded following publication of this book. Nonetheless, the influence of the profit motive seems likely to remain stable.

Entrepreneurial success is associated with drive and innovation. I have observed, however, that profitable health care companies and institutions, accountable to strong external regulation, become inherently conservative. Understandably, they want to stay with a winning approach and maximize profits. This strategy often has a dampening effect on creativity of rehabilitation professionals, since holistic and occupationally based programs would use less routine and more individualized methods. Unless these methods were carefully documented to emphasize functional outcomes, reimbursement might be questioned. Therefore, perceived financial risk frequently discourages a holistic approach to occupational therapy practice.

Intrinsic norms in these settings protect profitable procedures. They explicitly and implicitly encourage therapists to

- Do, don't talk
- Take the shortest route to a measurable goal
- Perform services that have been reimbursed before
- Document only standard treatment modalities
- Quantify outcomes and avoid qualitative data
- Move on to the next patient as quickly as possible.

These norms are so embedded in some rehabilitation settings that some therapists no longer notice their insidious impact on the quality of practice and on job satisfaction.

Much to their credit, many occupational therapists have managed to preserve collaborative, holistic approaches to functional rehabilitation in geriatric treatment settings. There are administrators and agencies whose values are congruent with such an approach. It is notable that a strong emphasis has emerged on the improvement of function. Where function is the focus, occupation becomes important, and purpose and meaning in activity achieve value beyond the simple quantity of performances.

The next chapter of this book will describe a holistic approach to geriatric occupational therapy treatment. Here are a few ideas about restoring a holistic basis for practice in the clinical culture discussed above.

In my experience, it does not require additional time to discuss patients' life stories during and after initial evaluation. Talking and doing can be interspersed in an evaluation or treatment setting. A reasonable rhythm of activity and rest is a benefit to the treatment of older adults. Discussion often creates the motivation for action. Discovering what a person likes to do can translate to an occupational plan for the following session. Collaborating with the patient in this way means that the therapist need not waste time trying to come up with an appropriate occupational focus.

Occupational performance can be documented in measurable terms. It is frequently more cost effective than standard exercises or modalities, because the patient is performing the very occupations he or she wishes to pursue in daily life. Assistance levels and progress are clear. The patient need not transfer learning or functional skills to a new task if he or she has been working with the desired occupation all along.

With careful selection, a therapist can complete a few successful, well-documented, and reimbursed treatments using a holistic occupational approach. Administrative support then might develop to identify frequent occupational interests among the patient population, order relevant supplies, and include motivational and historical factors in the evaluation format.

As therapists incorporate discussion and occupation with other treatment modalities, other disciplines gradually accommodate to a modified occupational therapy role. Some discussions and negotiations may be necessary for a positive outcome in this regard. Finally, a program of cost-effective and relevant groups can evolve as the rehabilitation team becomes comfortable with a collaborative, holistic model.

AN INTERACTIVE RESOURCE FOR CLINICIANS AND STUDENTS

A high and increasing proportion of occupational therapists work with elders (Peterson, Bergstone, & Douglass, 1988). Specialized education in gerontology is considered necessary for therapists to recognize the complex developmental, health, and occupational needs of clients in this practice area (Hasselkus & Kiernat, 1989). A survey of 101 occupational therapy programs found that a majority required course work in human development and gerontology (Stone & Martens, 1991). Only 53 percent, however, specifically addressed the issue of patient motivation and compliance with treatment suggestions. Fifty-six percent included information about autonomy and choice of activities in institutions. Forty-three percent discussed occupational therapy consultation to activity programming. Many new graduates, therefore, are unevenly trained in these subject areas.

Clinical supervision is a potential avenue to improve the preparation and abilities of therapists. Unfortunately, the culture of supervision seems quite weak in geriatric rehabilitation, given the complexity of practice. In acute care and subacute settings, time pressures, documentation requirements, and profit margins create strong disincentives to regular, in-depth supervision meetings. In the burgeoning home-care area, geographic separation of itinerant therapists compounds the problem. It is notable that occupational therapy practice with long-term-care patients is limited to brief forays for improving specific functional skills. Few resources exist to assist therapists treating older, developmentally delayed patients (Lowe, 1995).

The lack of consistent, strong supervision may contribute to practitioners' concentration on technical aspects of treatment and may impede their professional development. West (1990) insists that principles rather than techniques, and knowledge rather than skills, are needed for practitioners to become creative in identifying and solving clinical problems.

According to Frum and Opacich (1987), good supervision can help students and therapists move from a state of stagnation and confusion to one of integration, characterized by flexible, creative thinking. Frum and Opacich credit ongoing supervision with strengthening therapists' ability to make autonomous decisions, translate knowledge into purposeful action, monitor their own motivations and emotional responses, and develop a personal frame of reference and ethical standards.

Mattingly (1994) states that occupational therapy bridges two cultures: the biomedical culture, which emphasizes disease, and the culture of professions, such as social work, psychology, and pastoral counseling, which addresses the illness experience. Therefore, occupational therapists must work toward physiological, functional goals, and toward goals that involve coping and adaptation. Clinical reasoning studies in our field have found that therapists often shift uneasily in their thinking between these two cultural approaches or "tracks," even in a single session.

It is the editor's intention to provide concepts, information, and case material that will encourage self-reflection, supervision, and flexible clinical reasoning. These elements are indispensable for mature and expert professional practice in occupational therapy.

REFERENCES

American Association of Retired Persons & Administration on Aging. (1990). *A profile of older Americans.* Washington, D.C.: Authors.

AOTA PAC (1995, June 29). Call to action: Occupational therapists urged to contact congress. *OT Week,* 12–13.

Beers, M., & Urice, S. (1992). *Aging in good health.* New York: Pocket Books.

Berthelette, M., & Lewis, C. (1995, July 3). Are occupational therapists still the function experts? *OT Advance, 2,* 15.

Billig, N. (1993). *Growing older and wiser.* New York: Macmillan.

Bonder, B. (1993). Issues in assessment of psychosocial components of function. *American Journal of Occupational Therapy, 47,* 211–216.

Bonder, B. (1994). The psychosocial meaning of activity. In B. Bonder & M. Wagner (Eds.), *Functional performance in older adults.* Philadelphia: F.A. Davis.

Carlson, M., Fanchiang, S., Zemke, R., & Clark, F. (1996). A meta-analysis of the effectiveness of occupational therapy services for older persons. *American Journal of Occupational Therapy, 50,* 89–98.

Christenson. (1995). Conference on Aging: Its Impact on Occupational Therapy. *OT Week, 9*(23), 26-27.

Clark, C., Corcoran, M., & Gitlin, L. (1995). An exploratory study of how occupational therapists develop therapeutic relationships with family caregivers. *American Journal of Occupational Therapy, 49,* 587–594.

Cohen, G. (1993). Foreword. In N. Billig (Ed.), *Growing older and wiser.* New York: Macmillan.

Coleman, P. (1984). Assessing self-esteem and its sources in elderly people. *Aging and Society, 4,* 117–135.

Collen, M. (1993). Better health care for the elderly. In F. Lieberman & M. Collen (Eds.), *Aging in good health: A quality lifestyle for the later years.* New York: Plenum.

Evans, W., & Rosenberg, I. (1991). *Biomarkers: The ten determinants of aging you can control.* New York: Simon & Schuster

Felts, W. (1993). Cost-effective health care for the elderly: An internist's perspective. In F. Lieberman & M. Collen (Ed.), *Aging in good health: A quality lifestyle for the later years.* New York: Plenum.

Friedland, J., & Renwick, R. (1993). Psychosocial occupational therapy: Time to cast off the gloom and doom. *American Journal of Occupational Therapy, 47,* 467–471.

Frum, D., & Opacich, K. (1987). *Supervision: Development of therapeutic competence.* Bethesda, MD: American Occupational Therapy Association.

Hasselkus, B., & Kiernat, J. (1989). Nationally speaking: Not by age alone: Gerontology as a specialty in occupational therapy. *American Journal of Occupational Therapy, 43,* 77–79.

Helfrich, C., Kielhofner, G., & Mattingly, C. (1994). Volition as narrative: Understanding motivation in chronic illness. *American Journal of Occupational Therapy, 48,* 311–317.

Kern, S. (1994). In L. Marmer, Insurers, OTs on opposite edges of philosophical chasm. *OT Advance, 10,* 14–15.

Lazarus, L., Newton, N., Cohle, R., et al. (1987). Frequency and presentation of depressive symptoms in patients with primary degenerative dementia. *American Journal of Psychiatry, 114,* 41.

Levine, R., & Gitlin, L. (1993). A model to promote activity competence in elders. *American Journal of Occupational Therapy, 47,* 147–153.

Lowe, H. (1995, July 10). To the editor: Adult developmental disabilities programming being overlooked. *OT Advance, 2,* 3.

Mattingly, C. (1994). Occupational therapy as a two-body practice. In C. Mattingly & M. Hayes (Eds.), *Clinical reasoning: Forms of inquiry in a therapeutic practice.* Philadelphia: F.A. Davis.

Neistadt, M., & Seymour, S. (1995). Treatment activity preferences of occupational therapists in adult physical dysfunction settings. *American Journal of Occupational Therapy, 49,* 437–443.

Ory, M., & Williams, T. (1989, May). Rehabilitation: Small goals, sustained interventions. *Annals of the American Academy of Political and Social Science, 503,* 60–71.

Pearson, D., & Shaw, S. (1982). *Life extension.* New York: Warner Books.

Pelland, M. (1987). A conceptual model for the instruction and supervision of treatment planning. *American Journal of Occupational Therapy, 41,* 351–359.

Peloquin, S. (1990). The patient–therapist relationship in occupational therapy: Understanding visions and images. *American Journal of Occupational Therapy, 44,* 13–21.

Peterson, D., Bergstone, D., & Douglass, E. (1988). *Employment in the field of aging: The supply and demand in four professions.* Los Angeles: University of Southern California and Association for Gerontology in Higher Education.

Stone, R., & Martens, K. (1991). Educating entry-level occupational therapy students in gerontology. *American Journal of Occupational Therapy, 45*, 643–650.

Taylor, E., & Manguno, J. (1991). Use of treatment activities in occupational therapy. *American Journal of Occupational Therapy, 45*, 317–322.

Versluys, H. (1995). Evaluation of emotional adjustment to disabilities. In C. Trombly (Ed.), *Occupational therapy for physical dysfunction* (4th ed., pp. 225–234). Baltimore: Williams & Wilkins.

West, W. (1990). Nationally speaking—perspectives on the past and future, Part 2. *American Journal of Occupational Therapy, 44*, 9–10.

White House Conference on Aging. (1995, May). Washington, DC: Authors.

Yerxa, E., & Sharrott, G. (1986). Liberal arts: The foundation for occupational therapy education. *American Journal of Occupational Therapy, 40*, 153–159.

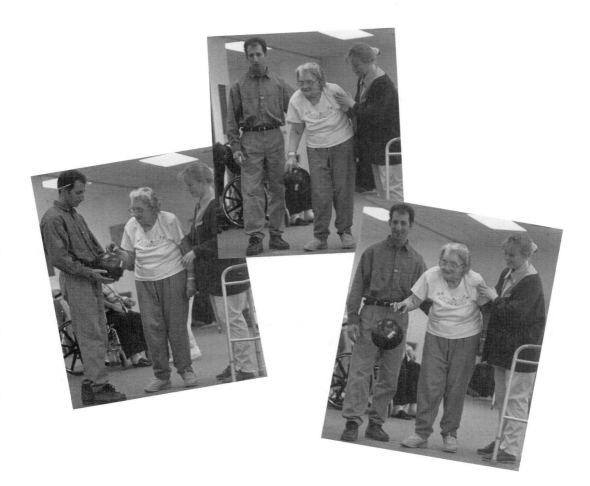

Chapter 2 *Theory and Practice in Evaluation and Treatment*

Mark S. Rosenfeld, PhD, OTR/L

THE THREADS OF EXISTENCE

Isaac Bashevis Singer (1953) writes about a little old shoemaker in Eastern Europe with a long family history in his trade. During World War II, his wife is killed, his home is burned, and his town is destroyed. The shoemaker wanders across Europe like a sleepwalker, stunned and confused. When found by his children, he is ragged, weak, and disoriented. They fear he will die. One day, in his confusion, the shoemaker stumbles into a closet and finds the tools of his trade, which he carried in his bag from home. Automatically, he picks up a shoe and begins to work. The songs once sung at his workbench spring again to his lips. Soon he is repairing all the shoes in the neighborhood. His strength and awareness return, to the delight of his family.

This story begins with a profound disruption to the life context of an individual. It ends with the restoration of health and relationships. The shoemaker rises to the cues of his familiar tools. Habituated responses are activated.

Abilities, role performance, and identity are gradually reclaimed as the threads of existence are rewoven in a new context. This is an occupational therapy parable, to be sure.

The Torn Threads: Sudden Illness and Injury

The onset of severe illness or injury is a crisis-precipitating event disrupting the life contexts of elderly patients. Like the shoemaker, older adults in a medical crisis are in danger of losing a great deal. Life itself is often threatened, and the future is fearful and clouded. Independence and autonomy are compromised. Admission to a hospital or nursing home is a wrenching separation from the past, and from home, neighborhood, and relationships. The possibility exists that one will never return to familiar surroundings and to people who know one's identity, family, and life achievements. In such an environment, the sense of belonging is lost.

In subacute rehabilitation practice, I regularly meet people in crisis, struggling with such problems. At first glance, I see a portrait of each person at a difficult moment in life. Every individual responds differently to disability. I cannot predict rehabilitation outcome, therefore, from knowledge of medical diagnosis alone. I must understand the portrait beneath, the pentimento of past life, family, and accomplishment to find the avenues and the potential for rehabilitation. Life context connects us with this world; and preserving that connection is the motivating force for treatment. It is no wonder that many institutionalized elders wait longingly for visitors and express no desire more strongly than to go home.

Medical Crisis and Occupational Intervention

Dixon (1987) states that each crisis has a nucleus, a *nuclear problem*, that threatens something the person considers essential for meaningful life. Occupational therapists, I believe, must understand that problem and find the *nuclear tasks*, the critical things that need doing to resolve the crisis. The right tasks reestablish a sense of continuity in life by drawing from the individual's past and actively creating future possibilities. The right tasks mobilize the person to accept the challenge of his or her situation, to try, and to succeed, despite the pain and frustration involved (Rosenfeld, 1984). The specific functions of nuclear tasks are to *express* and manage feelings, *sustain* occupational patterns and involvements, *learn* vital new skills, *remotivate* by demonstrating self-reliance, and *symbolize* recovery.

I recently encountered a woman in her late 80s, who suffers from dementia, sitting in a busy hallway at a nursing home. She was reaching toward passers-

by, crying out that she did not know where she was. She repeated the seemingly rhetorical question, "What can I do now?" As an occupational therapist, I take that question literally. I stopped, introduced myself, and acknowledged the woman's upset. I asked her what she had enjoyed doing in the past. "I used to knit afghans all the time," she remembered. After a trip to the supply closet, we sat in the same busy hallway and knitted. The woman's face cleared of tears and anxiety. Organized and absorbed, she patiently taught me, a rank beginner, the basic stitch. A half-hour later, the woman discussed her business school education and her 35 years as a bookkeeper for the family business. We made plans for her to help with clerical tasks in the Rehabilitation Department.

While dementing illness is by no means cured by such intervention, the emotional crisis it caused is moderated. Knitting, in this example, is a sustaining activity since it continues a positive occupational pattern disrupted by crisis events. It is a remotivating activity as well, since it clearly demonstrates to the woman, to me, and to all observers, her competence. Its performance reminds her of other areas of competence and accomplishment in her life as well. This activity is also symbolic of a move toward recovery of self-control, of ability, and of identity. It is a mile marker in a long race.

No doubt, this patient will forget her success by the following day. No matter; we have found the necessary nuclear tasks and can return to them at will. Many nuclear tasks involve learning new skills. Physical rehabilitation requires intensive effort in this regard. Many elderly patients work hard to recapture functional abilities that they need to live a more satisfying life.

Retieing the Threads: Integrating Function, Purpose, and Life Context in Treatment

ADL, functional mobility, upper extremity exercise, and safety skills training may be the hardware of geriatric occupational therapy practice. But motivation for treatment is the software; and motivation is embedded in the life history, character, values, and occupational experiences of the individual. Performing meaningful activities in treatment reassures patients that life context is not lost, that less is not necessarily meaningless, that there is hope. In a study of elderly patients, Zimmer-Branum and Nelson (1995) demonstrated strong patient preference for occupational forms as compared to straight exercise. Kircher (1984) found that subjects perceived less exertion while sustaining effort in performing purposeful (rope jumping) versus non-purposeful (jumping) activities.

Failing to understand the occupational history of our patients severely reduces our therapeutic resources. Ironically, many medical charts do not contain basic information about patients' occupational history beyond their recent living situation. If you are old and sick, many other facts about your life are considered unimportant by medical systems.

A colleague in a nursing home asked me to see a patient with Parkinson's disease one day. The patient had refused treatment the previous day, and the therapist complained that he was "so slow that he drove her crazy." No doubt the patient perceived this as well. The man was slow and methodical in performing upper extremity dressing and grooming activities. He took 15 minutes cleaning his electric razor. I learned that he had assembled complex and expensive electronics equipment during 46 years of employment. His extreme care in task performance was a valuable asset. By her ignorance, a therapist had transformed this strength into a weakness.

The occupational therapist's approach, the goals of treatment, and the selection of purposeful nuclear tasks rest on a holistic foundation. Such a framework has been widely supported in the occupational therapy literature (Crabtree, 1991; Fisher & Short-DeGraff, 1993; Friedland & Renwick, 1993; Haas, 1995; Kirkland & Davis, 1988; Mattingly & Flemming, 1994; Peloquin, 1990; Rogers, 1981; Versluys, 1995; Watson, 1986; Watts, Kielhofner, Bauer, Gregory, & Valentine, 1986). To implement a holistic treatment philosophy, therapists must create room for intense curiosity about their patients' lives. I believe we must recognize a person in order to restore one. Case examples follow in which the treatment integrates function, purpose, and life context.

In meeting a sad-looking 81-year-old widow who had arthritis and was legally blind, I inquired about the name of the stuffed cat she held. This led to tears about the loss of her real cat and her home the day she fell and broke her hip. The woman explained how hard she had worked to earn a living and raise her children as a single parent. Now, she despaired of seeing her family on Thanksgiving, the following day. In our session, we called her niece on the phone (mod assist) and confirmed an invitation for the holiday. Then we practiced safe transfers, motivated by the woman's worry about getting in and out of the car and house the next day. When we were done, I praised her spirit, her commitment to relationships, and her perseverance. By finding the purpose in functioning, we established a reason to try. We also addressed prescribed functional goals that included ADL retraining (telephone), functional mobility, and upper extremity exercise (transfer training), which totaled five units of billable service.

I was asked to work with an isolated 90-year-old woman with Parkinson's disease to improve motor skills. Her room was dark in midday, and she sat woodenly in the only chair. Looking for a place to sit, I inquired if the foot of the bed would be all right. Then I saw the flicker of a smile cross her face. I asked what amused her, and she replied, "It's been a long time since a man sat on my bed." "Gee, that's too bad," I responded. "How long has it been?" Our subsequent discussion about the role of love and romance in her life led the woman to remember and recognize her need for contact with others. Card games had been her favorite pastime. We played a few hands, for dexterity and concentration, of course. By the end of the day, I had found a card partner for her among the residents on her floor. Antidepressant medications and peg-board exercises cannot rehabilitate

as well as an occupational therapist. Rehabilitation occurs when function and meaning are integrated in the actions of an individual.

Nelson and Stucky (1992) state that effective occupational interventions present situations that are interesting and purposeful, make sense to the person, are compatible with identity and world view, offer choices, make an impact on the environment, and require the person's efforts for completion. In nursing home settings, improvement in well-being and activity level of long-term residents is associated with therapeutic optimism of the staff, choices and control over the environment, and participation in purposeful activity programs (Joseph & Wanlass, 1993).

Surmounting Obstacles to a Holistic Approach

Many occupational therapists are more comfortable defining function than meaning. Fast-paced practice and narrow reimbursement guidelines have driven practice away from life context, from motivational issues, and from meaning in rehabilitation activities. Therapists often direct patients back to the functional task agenda when they "stray" into territory that involves meaning, history, hope, and life context. They close off critical communication just when enthusiastic curiosity would be desirable. Mattingly and Flemming (1994) found that a surface orientation to evaluation was taken by many therapists. The use of long functional checklists and rating scales frequently guaranteed that no problem area could be examined in depth.

There are several reasons for inattention to life context, meaning, and motivation. Therapists may consider these issues superfluous, outside their expertise, beyond occupational therapy's domain of concern, upsetting for the patient, unsettling for the therapist, or as obstacles to treatment. Others discuss these issues with their patients but feel guilty about doing so. Therapists are unclear about the connection of these discussions to the rehabilitation process. "We are paid to do, not to talk," they insist. Therefore, they do not document or bill directly for interventions to reduce psychosocial obstacles and improve motivation, even though these interventions are crucial to the entire treatment effort. These interventions can be tied directly to functional outcomes by demonstrating improvements in occupational performance or subcomponent skills.

Some therapists worry that recognizing a patient as I suggest is a time-consuming proposition. In my clinical experience, it takes no longer to address life history issues in concert with functional evaluation and treatment tasks than not to address the issues. Units of service are the same. It is the quality of care that is improved. Patients talk about their illness and life context issues because they need to tell their stories, share their burdens, reformulate their identities, and invent their futures.

While danger is one element of a crisis, opportunity is another. People in crisis can grow beyond homeostasis, learn new meanings and new skills, and break new developmental ground if they have an active coping orientation and

good support. A 71-year-old woman I treated following her injury and her husband's death in a car accident is an excellent example of growth under pressure. This woman also had a long history of depression. Following a stroke 5 years before, she had become extremely dependent upon her husband, even to comb her hair and brush her teeth. She angrily refused therapy for a week after admission. This woman was clearly in pain but unapproachable. Medicare was about to decertify her treatment.

I shut the door and addressed her pain directly, insisting that she could not keep it all inside and needed to allow some other shoulders to help her bear it. Following a tearful recounting of her losses, the woman wondered aloud whether she would be too burdensome to live with her daughter and her family in the future. This concern for the future served as a stimulus for us to work together to evaluate her actual functional abilities. We did some mobility and ADL assessments. The woman saw that improved practical skills could better her chances to live with or near her family in the future. After making some functional progress in treatment, the woman asked me how she ever had become so helpless and dependent. I shrugged, and we both had a good laugh.

All the treatment described above was legitimate and reimbursable occupational therapy. None of the functional gains would have occurred without the initial session that required a great deal of talking in order to establish a basis for doing.

THEORIES OF AGING, MOTIVATION, AND INTERVENTION

Old Age as a Life Stage

Approaches to aging as a developmental process vary. Some stress the relative proximity of death (Becker, 1973; DeBeauvoir, 1973) and the prevalence of losses (work role, spouse, income, physical frailty) as negative factors. An increased frequency of depression is cited among older adults (Coleman, 1984; Fassler & Gaviria, 1978). On the other hand, older people have been found to adjust to losses well (Bowling & Cartwright, 1982) and to have a higher level of life satisfaction as compared to their younger counterparts (Abrams, 1978). Certainly, we recognize that old age is as varied an experience as any other developmental stage.

Erikson's (1950) description of the tension between "ego-integrity" and "despair" seems to capture a thematic focus for the challenges of old age. High self-esteem is often seen as the linchpin of quality of life in old age (Coleman, 1984). The ability to perceive oneself in control of events is a critical factor in this regard (Rodin, 1986; Rogers, 1990). Frankl (1963) emphasized purpose in life, even small daily goals, as central to psychic integrity. Levine and Gitlin (1993) cited the ongoing importance of activity competence in older adults.

The prevalence of reminiscence among elders indicates a need to process life experiences (Stevens-Ratchford, 1993) and to retain a strong cognitive connection with the people, places, and events that compose one's life context

(Dunn, Brown, & McGuigan, 1994; Kielhofner, 1993). Reminiscence helps to support the value of "continuity theory" as a way to understand the motivational forces in old age (Atchley, 1989; Victor, 1988). Continuity theory suggests that we strive to maintain a close connection with our internal "cognitive map" of life (Taplin, 1971), which is lived out in the lifestyle we have shaped (Rosenfeld, 1993).

From an occupational therapy standpoint, then, a positive process of aging requires several elements. These elements include an active coping orientation in response to problems, the ability to deal with loss and change, formulation of clear and realistic personal goals, continued engagement with important people and activities, and positive self-evaluations regarding performance. While some disabled elders struggle mightily to restore continuity, others disengage. They lower their expectations, embrace dependency, and accept a shrinking and stultifying personal life space.

Illness and Injury as Threats to Life Continuity

The onset of severe disability is an extreme life-changing event in its impact on daily life, the future, and the need for ongoing adaptations. As a result, rehabilitation is a psychosocial process that goes far beyond issues of health per se (Kemp, 1990a). Ornish (1993) states that the word "heal" derives from a Greek root meaning "to make whole." It is recognized that illness can cause discontinuity and disruption in the cognitive map (Taplin, 1971) and life story (Helfrich,

Kielhofner, & Mattingly, 1994) of a human being.

As previously discussed, admission to a treatment facility brings additional threats to identity and integrity, which include lost abilities, increased dependency, decreased autonomy, and dislocation from social supports, familiar surroundings, valued activities, and personal routines (Hasselkus, 1978; Watson, 1986).

Many theorists have described stages of response to severe injury or illness (Fink, 1967; Hendrick, 1981; Kerr, 1977; Strain, Grossman, 1975; Vargo, 1978). Most theories recognize an initial period of shock or defensive retreat; the reality of events is too overwhelming to embrace. Gradually, oscillating between awareness and denial, the individual acknowledges the impact of illness or injury. This stage is marked by intense anger and sadness.

During shock and acknowledgment, according to Maslow (1970), safety needs are primary. A 90-year-old former operating room nurse once yelled at me when I asked her to practice a tub transfer. She insisted on an immediate discharge to home, despite her balance and safety problems. The woman could not, early in treatment, tolerate a demonstration of her incapacities, her need to rely on others. She had been capable and in charge for many years in her personal and professional life. I put her in charge of me and of our session that day. In response to anxiety about discharge, I clarified with nursing staff the estimated length of her stay and communicated this information to the patient. I asked her how I should help

her to check for safety in tub transfers, and she led me to the tub room to instruct me.

In the adjustment stage, growth needs emerge. A new outlook, new learning, and new skills are sought in efforts to adapt to disability and a changed life situation. This cycle does not usually occur in a singular or linear fashion. Rather, medical changes, new challenges, discharge from treatment, and a host of other events may cause the person to cycle back through the entire process again. Furthermore, individuals respond differently. As with all forms of severe adversity, some disabled people may become withdrawn and embittered, while others become more open and compassionate (Kushner, 1981). Disability may be perceived as an enemy, a punishment, a weakness, a challenge, a loss, or a relief of responsibility (Lipowski, 1970). A substantial number of people continue to enhance their abilities long after rehabilitation treatment ends. Many others lose functional ground quickly following discharge (Brummell-Smith, 1993).

Attitudinal stumbling blocks frequently interfere with rehabilitation (Hesse, Campion, & Karamouz, 1984). Due to ageism, the elderly may wrongly assume that progressive disability is inevitable. Some feel that longevity has earned them the right to be taken care of by others. Physical and emotional fatigue also inhibit energetic participation in the treatment process. Crisis theory provides a useful framework for viewing individual responses to disability (Dixon, 1987; Slaikeu, 1984). Onset of disability is a crisis-precipitating event when it presents a severe threat to something the person considers essential for identity or meaning in life. The person is presented with a nuclear problem that cannot be solved by normal means and is thrown into a 1–6 week period of confusion and emotional turmoil. Functioning plummets and disequilibrium prevails.

Although the symptoms of illness or injury may be the same for two individuals, the medical event or diagnosis can precipitate a crisis for one person and not the other. Hill (1965) explains that a crisis is defined by the precipitating event as it interacts with the meaning given to the event by the person, which in turn interacts with the crisis-meeting resources of that individual. These resources include social and material supports, and coping abilities.

Crisis = Precipitating Event <—> Meaning Given to Event <—> Crisis-Meeting Resources

To surmount the crisis, in theory, the person must perceive the challenge inherent in the situation, not simply the threat or the loss. While threat and loss lead to anxiety and depression, challenge mobilizes the person to take active steps, problem solve, and cope. In this respect, a crisis presents both a danger and an opportunity.

The danger includes adoption of maladaptive coping patterns and the permanent loss of function in life. Substance abuse, impulsive or passive behavior, and ongoing emotion spilling are common responses. These patterns are quickly learned because they temporarily reduce anxiety, although they produce negative consequences as well.

The opportunity during crisis is for maturation and growth beyond former levels. People are often open to change and to influence during a crisis, when their usual ways of coping are inadequate to reduce tension, restore equilibrium, and resolve the troubling situation. Therefore, crisis presents a golden opportunity for intervention (Dixon, 1987; Slaikeu, 1984).

Hill's research (1965) suggests that a history of success in handling adversity can predict success in surmounting a current crisis, and that failure in the past predicts failure as well. Occupational therapists recognize that immediate success in tackling rehabilitation tasks and learning new skills can mediate and even reverse this rather fatalistic correlation (Rosenfeld, 1984). Clearly, motivation, action, and self-assessment are crucial variables.

Motivational Issues in Rehabilitation

Occupational therapists are consistently asked to determine the rehabilitation potential of patients in order to justify expenditures for skilled services. Motivation for treatment occupies a central position among many variables that bear on this potential. Perceived lack of motivation contributes to the early decertification of many elderly rehabilitation candidates (Hesse et al., 1984).

Kemp (1990b) reports that factors associated with rehabilitation success include: patient assertiveness, goal directedness, and presence of an intimate relationship. Factors associated with rehabilitation failure include poor motivation, cognitive impairment (i.e., Mini Mental Status Exam score below 22), depression, passivity, dependency, hysteria, and a suspicious approach to relationships in treatment. Recognizing the complexity of the issue, Mosqueda (1993) argues that physical, cognitive, psychological, social, and economic perspectives of a patient's condition and resources are vital to the assessment of rehabilitation potential.

Rehabilitation can be a difficult process. It requires that a disabled older adult endure pain and devote precious energies to perform hard work, which is sometimes repetitive and boring. Positive results are not consistent, one's inabilities are graphically evident, and indignities are frequent. Therefore, motivation is the most important problem facing the rehabilitation professional (Fishman, 1962). To foster motivation, therapists must be effective psychosocial advocates as well as functional coaches. Practitioners are just beginning to develop systematic methods to evaluate and enhance motivation in rehabilitation settings (Brummell-Smith, 1993).

According to Miller and Rollnick (1991), motivation is not a personality trait. Rather, it is an internal state influenced by external factors. While physical surroundings, equipment, supplies, and activities are central to rehabilitation efforts, relationships are considered crucial. The existence and involvement of a significant other have been found to predict rehabilitation success. The therapist can provide an important relationship in the treatment milieu and influence patient motivation as well

(Baum, 1980; King, 1980; Peloquin, 1990). A therapist's style can have a significant impact in a single session (Miller & Sovereign, 1989). Empathy and reflective listening clarify and amplify a patient's experience and meaning related to illness, treatment, and recovery.

Rosenfeld (1990) suggested that a therapeutic contact in occupational therapy moves systematically from reflecting to planning to doing in a measured sequence. Miller and Rollnick (1991) describe this process as similar to improvisational theater. Each patient and therapist proceed differently. The therapist must carefully match his or her approach to the patient's need for contemplation, determination to change, planning, or action, for therapy to succeed. The authors warn that standard programs eliminate crucial opportunities for patients to feel freedom and exert responsibility in making treatment choices. This reduces the likelihood that the individual will enter into, continue with, and adhere to a specific change strategy or plan. Mattingly and Flemming (1994) and Fidler (1995) also advocate individualizing treatment activities by tailoring them to the specific skills, needs, and interests of the patient. This approach mobilizes the person to action.

It is positive action on the part of the patient that indicates the presence of "motivation" and that creates functional improvements in treatment outcomes. Joiner and Hansel (1996) conclude that treatment facilities often disempower clients by making decisions about eating, sleeping, scheduling, and treatment modalities for them. Joiner and Hansel argue for client empowerment through joint problem solving, decision making, and explicit contracting for treatment.

Despite a strong emphasis on patient collaboration in the literature, Neistadt (1995) and Northen, Rust, Nelson, and Watts (1995) found that occupational therapists who work with patients with physical dysfunction do not maximize patient participation in treatment decisions. Therapists miss opportunities to elicit and clarify patient goals, expectations, and occupational preferences. In Fidler's view (1992), lack of patient involvement can weaken a milieu and inhibit strivings for autonomy, independence, improved performance, relationships, and occupational satisfaction.

Family members' lives are powerfully affected by the need to care for a disabled relative (Bahr & Peterson, 1989). Family members are crucial participants in the process of adjustment to disability. Their struggles, needs, and motivations must be carefully considered if rehabilitation plans are to succeed. Clark, Corcoran, and Gitlin (1995) suggest that therapists must shift from simply informing and directing caregivers, toward caring and partnering with them. This approach reduces the likelihood that rehabilitation plans will fail due to patients, therapists, and caregivers pulling in different directions.

Kemp (1990b) offers a helpful equation regarding motivation for rehabilitation. He cautions that motivation can vary in effort and in direction (for or against the process). The factors that shape motivation include the patient's

wants, beliefs, and *rewards.* Since motivational influences are highly individual, they must be carefully appraised.

Wants consist of the goals and desires held by the person for recovery, improved functioning, return to the community, or a desired living environment. These wants are the driving forces for treatment. Without them, rehabilitation activities have no purpose in the patient's mind. A 90-year-old woman in considerable discomfort confided in me that she wished to die. She had a dream, she explained, in which Jesus appeared before her and affixed beautiful wings to her back. While she had enjoyed her life, the dream focused her yearnings toward a heavenly peace. Although functional restoration was not this patient's primary concern, she worked in therapy so that she could return home. To die in familiar surroundings at her appointed time was a meaningful objective.

Beliefs frame the patient's understanding of the medical situation, expectations regarding prognosis, and rehabilitation treatment. Clearly, there must be a belief in the possibility for improvement if treatment participation is to be meaningful. It should not be assumed that patients have an accurate understanding of their prognoses or of rehabilitation potential and procedures. Frequently, depression colors patients' wants and beliefs. Hopelessness, decreased concentration, anhedonia, and psychomotor retardation weaken participation and performance of rehabilitation tasks. In some instances, psychostimulant medications such as Ritalin, Cylert, and Dexedrine may be particularly helpful in rapidly energizing depressed patients (Weintraub, 1995). These medicines have a low morbidity rate. Antidepressant medications (tricyclics and selective serotonin reuptake inhibitors) may take several weeks to work. The use of rapid-acting psychostimulants can help patients to participate productively while funding for valuable and limited treatment time is available.

The *rewards* of rehabilitation are sometimes clear and accessible. Evidence of progress, opportunities for participation in valued occupations, and discharge to an improved life situation are powerful reinforcers. Kemp (1990b) points out, however, that these rewards are inconsistent and sometimes inadequate to sustain motivation. In these instances, extrinsic rewards may be necessary.

An 80-year-old woman with a fractured tibia, for example, complained she was too tired when I arrived for her session. "Can't we skip today?" she asked. "Why don't you drive me somewhere in your car instead?" I refused, but asked where she would go, given the opportunity. "Somewhere entertaining," she said. "A stand-up comedy place would be good, cause I could use a laugh." I insisted we have our therapy session, but arranged a video showing of a Honeymooner's bloopers tape immediately to follow. Having the good laugh she wanted made the hard work worth the effort.

Rogers (1990) asserts that perceived self-competence determines a patient's efforts and satisfaction in the rehabilitation process. Since people differ widely in their ways of explaining success and failure (their attributional style) (Fayans, 1980), therapists must carefully observe the judgments patients make about their performance and progress. Negotiation and reality testing are often necessary in this regard.

An older woman with a hip fracture, for example, made slow but steady progress in her rehabilitation. Despite improvements, however, she always focused on how much she still could not do. Her discouragement diminished her energy and effort. I pointed out her "glass half empty" way of seeing things. The woman readily admitted this but felt she could not change. With a contract to try, with persistent monitoring and substitution of more positive cognitions and statements, the patient was able to describe and to feel "the glass half full." "I just need a little assistance with the last 6 inches down to sitting, now," she said. "Six weeks ago, I needed two people to carry me from the wheelchair to the toilet!" Her affect and her efforts improved.

The major detracting factors in motivation are the *costs* of rehabilitation. These include, pain, energy expenditure, risk, frustration, and the indignity and shame of imperfect performance. For many patients, illness has mobilized caretakers to spend time with them and look after their needs. Such care and dependency can be quite seductive. It is important to recognize that rehabilitation leads to a loss of help and support as abilities and independence are restored. No wonder that discharge from occupational therapy often stimulates feelings of sadness and anxiety as well as accomplishment. The costs of rehabilitation treatment must be assessed and mediated for each patient, if motivation for treatment is to persist. Kemp's (1990b) equation is as follows:

$$\text{Motivation} = \frac{\text{Wants} \times \text{Beliefs} \times \text{Rewards}}{\text{Costs}}$$
direction
effort

Based on a review of literature on rehabilitation potential, I consolidated salient factors into five categories and formatted them for a rating scale. (See chapter 12 for more detail.) The categories address the patient's health status, occupational and coping history, hopefulness, response to available support, and goal-directed performance. A content validity study with therapists in subacute treatment settings (n = 30) (Van Etten, 1995) and another with therapists, patients, and healthy elders (n = 126) (Breidel et al., 1995) affirmed the relevance of these factors. It is notable that the health status variables were given least saliency by the therapists among the five categories. One might expect health status to be seen as most important by health professionals. Rather, clinicians increasingly emphasized psychosocial factors over medical factors as their years of experience increased.

Erikson (1976) described a devastating flood that undermined the sense of community among survivors of five towns. The disaster caused a cultural slide along several axes of variation among the affected population in West Virginia. Physically hardy and capable miners, for example, fell prey to illness, substance abuse, somatic complaints,

and apathy. As financial claims were settled and communities were rebuilt, many survivors returned to their former vitality, while others suffered more permanent losses.

Erikson's concept of situational shifts in capacity can be applied to older patients in occupational therapy treatment. Patient ratings for rehabilitation potential, therefore, should not be seen as fixed indicators. Rather, the ratings reflect current status along movable axes of variation. Just as a patient's potential can be reduced by increasing morbidity and other situational factors, so can it be improved by the therapeutic process and milieu. In addition to the value of rating current status, therefore, the scale can assist therapists in identifying obstacles to motivation and rehabilitation potential, which may be positively influenced through intervention.

CONCRETE STEPS FOR MOTIVATIONAL INTERVENTIONS

A holistic approach to occupational therapy intervention must embrace a broad context for evaluation and treatment. In concert with functional evaluation, I have found the following procedures to be valuable:

◆ Help the patient express and manage emotional upset related to injury, illness, and admission. Ask the patient how he or she is feeling. Identify and address immediate concerns, taking action based on the patient's priorities and needs. Concern, responsiveness, and collaborative effort in the first few minutes sets the tone and structure for all future treatment.

◆ Invite the patient to recount recent events related to illness, injury, or hospitalization. The story of a traumatic event needs to be told many times to be integrated and mastered. Acknowledge the intensity of the experience, positive coping efforts, and strong character traits demonstrated by the patient. Recognizing realistic strengths at a time of profound weakness and vulnerability mobilizes the patient to keep healthy and active abilities in operation and challenges negative, global self-perceptions caused by disability. Telling meaningful fragments of their life stories often helps patients to define and locate themselves in the past, present, and future.

◆ Formulate the nuclear problem (the meaning of the precipitating event and disability to the person), coping resources, and available supports. When appropriate, explain your understanding of the problem and seek the patient's corroboration or contradiction of your perspective. Understanding a troubling situation is an important component for mastery. Caplan (1964) identifies cognitive clarity about a crisis situation as one of the preconditions for its resolution.

◆ Strengthen identity and life context compromised by disability. Bring discussion of the patient's important people, places, and events into the treatment process. Review life accomplishments, roles, values, faiths, pleasures, regrets, and losses. Such discussions and activity foci retie the threads of life broken by illness and institutionalization. These discussions

clarify the "wants" or goals of the patient and strengthen in his or her mind the prospects for life continuity. Also, the modalities and motivation for treatment embedded in this material become evident.

◆ Assess patient motivation. Address the wants, beliefs, rewards, and costs perceived by the individual. Formulate a profile of the patient along the axes of rehabilitation potential: health status, history, hope, help, and health efforts. Make concerted efforts to improve the patient's status in specific areas that threaten the viability of treatment. Health status and coping history may not be changed. The patient's hopes, ability to accept help and collaborate, and his or her goal-directed actions and self-evaluations, however, are more open to influence. Open communication about the therapeutic relationship and the effectiveness of treatment is essential.

◆ Promote the patient's realistic appraisal of medical and rehabilitation possibilities. Recognize the uncertainties and the challenges ahead. Stress the impact of personal effort on outcome in the treatment process. Invite the patient to articulate goals for treatment and for life after discharge. Discuss concrete ADL objectives and broader life roles. Help the patient recognize that less is not necessarily meaningless.

◆ Define the specific challenges of rehabilitation with the patient. Promote active coping and learning. Foster realistic performance and progress appraisal. Maximize rewards and minimize costs of rehabilitation by flexibly negotiating and collaborating regarding treatment tasks and schedules. Feedback and reinforcement are strategic therapeutic tools.

◆ Select and implement a program of nuclear tasks. Some of these tasks can restore personal integrity while others help to restore functional and bodily integrity. As previously explained, occupational therapists select activities and interactions that help patients in *expressing* and managing painful feelings; in *sustaining* performance of previously beneficial occupations and routines; in *learning new skills* for functional improvement, communication, stress management, and safety; in *symbolizing* progress toward recovery; or that are *remotivating* by demonstrating the person's ability to accomplish goals and take care of himself or herself.

While occupational therapy treatment plans often focus on the development or restoration of functional skills, the actual domain of concern reflected in treatment is much broader. Performance of nuclear tasks can be tied to practical functional outcomes and documented accordingly. If properly done, such documentation facilitates reimbursement for valuable, holistic interventions tied to the meaningful life context of the patient. This approach strengthens the broad, holistic framework for occupational therapy practice in gerontology.

REFERENCES

Abrams, M. (1978). Beyond three-score and ten: A first report on a survey of the elderly. *Age Concern England*. Surrey: Mitcham.

Atchley, R. (1989). Continuity theory of normal aging. *Gerontologist, 29*, 183.

Bahr, S., & Peterson, E. (1989). *Aging and the family*. Lexington, MA: Lexington Books.

Baum, C. (1980). Occupational therapists put care in the health system. *American Journal of Occupational Therapy, 34*, 505–516.

Becker, E. (1973). *The denial of death*. New York: Macmillan.

Bowling, A., & Cartwright, A. (1982). *Life after a death: A study of the elderly widowed*. London: Tavistock.

Breidel, D., Donoian, A., Landry, C., Parandes, K., Rock, D., Seiden, A., & Tarwog, N. (1995). *A measure of rehabilitation potential*. Unpublished study. Worcester, MA: Worcester State College.

Brummel-Smith, K. (1993). Research in rehabilitation. *Geriatric Rehabilitation, 9*, 895–904.

Caplan, G. (1964). *Principles of preventive psychiatry*. New York: Basic Books.

Clark, C., Corcoran, M., & Gitlin, L. (1995). An exploratory study of how occupational therapists develop therapeutic relationships with family caregivers. *American Journal of Occupational Therapy, 49*, 587–594.

Coleman, P. (1984). Assessing self-esteem and its sources in elderly people. *Aging and Society, 4*, 117–135.

Crabtree, J. (1991). Occupational therapy's new mandate: Providing services to the elderly. *American Journal of Occupational Therapy, 45*, 583–584.

DeBeauvoir, S. (1973). *A very easy death*. New York: Warner Books.

Dixon, S. (1987). *Working with people in crisis* (2nd ed.). St. Louis: Mosby.

Dunn, W., Brown, C., & McGuigan, A. (1994). The ecology of human performance: A framework for considering the effect of context. *American Journal of Occupational Therapy, 48*, 595–607.

Erikson, E. (1950). *Childhood and society*. New York: Norton.

Erikson, K. (1976). *Everything in its path*. New York: Simon & Schuster.

Fassler, L., & Gaviria, M. (1978). Depression in old age. *Journal of the American Geriatric Society, 26*, 471.

Fayans, L. (Ed.). (1980). *Achievement motivation*. New York: Plenum.

Fidler, G. (1992). *Recapturing competence: A system's change for geropsychiatric care*. New York: Springer.

Fidler, G. (1995). Position paper: The psychosocial core of occupational therapy. *American Journal of Occupational Therapy, 49,* 1021–1022.

Fink, S. (1967). Crisis and motivation: A theoretical model. *Archives of Physical Medicine and Rehabilitation, 48,* 592–597.

Fisher, A., & Short-DeGraff, M. (1993). Improving functional assessment in occupational therapy: Recommendations and philosophy for change. *American Journal of Occupational Therapy, 47,* 199–201.

Fishman, S. (1962). Amputation. In J. Garrett & E. Levine (Eds.), *Psychological practices with the physically disabled* (pp. 362–381). New York: Columbia University Press.

Frankl, V. (1963). *Man's search for meaning.* New York: Pocket Books.

Friedland, J., & Renwick, E. (1993). Psychosocial occupational therapy: Time to cast off the gloom and doom. *American Journal of Occupational Therapy, 47,* 467–471.

Haas, B. (1995). Clinical interpretation of "occupationally embedded exercise versus rote exercise: A choice between occupational forms by elderly nursing home residents." *American Journal of Occupational Therapy, 49,* 403–404.

Hasselkus, B. (1978). Relocation stress and the elderly. *American Journal of Occupational Therapy, 32,* 631–636.

Helfrich, C., Kielhofner, G., & Mattingly, C. (1994). Volition as narrative: Understanding motivation in chronic illness. *American Journal of Occupational Therapy, 48,* 311–317.

Hendrick, S. (1981, February). Spinal cord injury: A special kind of loss. *Personnel and Guidance Journal, 59,* 355–359.

Hesse, K., Campion, E., & Karamouz, N. (1984). Attitudinal stumbling blocks to geriatric rehabilitation. *Journal of the American Geriatric Society, 32,* 747.

Hill, R. (1965). Generic features of families under stress. In H. Parad (Ed.), *Crisis intervention: Selected readings,* (pp. 32–52). New York: Family Service Association of America.

Joiner, C., & Hansel, M. (1996). Empowering the geriatric client. *Occupational Therapy Practice, 1,* 34–39.

Joseph, C., & Wanlass, W. (1993). Rehabilitation in the nursing home. *Geriatric Rehabilitation, 9,* 859–871.

Kemp, B. (1990a). The psychosocial context of geriatric rehabilitation. In B. Kemp, K. Brunnell-Smith, & J. Ramsdell (Eds.), *Geriatric Rehabilitation* (pp. 41–57). Boston: College-Hill.

Kemp, B. (1990b). Motivational dynamics in geriatric rehabilitation: Toward a therapeutic model. In B. Kemp, K. Brunnell-Smith, & J. Ramsdell (Eds.), *Geriatric rehabilitation* (pp. 295–306). Boston: College-Hill.

Kerr, N. (1977). Understanding the process of adjustment to disability. In J. Stubbins (Ed.), *Social and psychological aspects of disability.* Baltimore: University Park Press.

Kielhofner, G. (1993). Functional assessment: Toward a dialectical view of person- environmental relations. *American Journal of Occupational Therapy, 47,* 248–251.

King, L.J. (1980). Creative caring. *American Journal of Occupational Therapy, 34,* 522–528.

Kircher, M. (1984). Motivation as a factor of perceived exertion in purposeful versus nonpurposeful activity. *American Journal of Occupational Therapy, 38,* 165–170.

Kirkland, M., & Davis, L. (Eds.). (1988). *ROTE manual: The role of occupational therapy with the elderly.* Bethesda, MD: American Occupational Therapy Association.

Kushner, H. (1981). *When bad things happen to good people.* New York: Avon Books.

Levine, R., & Gitlin, L. (1993). A model to promote activity competence in elders. *American Journal of Occupational Therapy, 47,* 147–153.

Lipowski, Z. (1970). Physical illness: The individual and the coping process. *International Journal of Psychiatry in Medicine, 1*(2), 98.

Maslow, A. (1970). *Motivation and personality* (2nd ed.). New York: Harper & Row.

Mattingly, C., & Flemming, M. (1994). *Clinical reasoning: Forms of inquiry in a therapeutic practice.* Philadelphia: F.A. Davis.

Miller, W., & Rollnick, S. (1991). *Motivational interviewing: Preparing people to change addictive behaviors.* New York: Guilford.

Miller, W., & Sovereign, R. (1989). The checkup: A model for early intervention in addictive behaviors. In T. Loberg, W. Miller, P. Nathan, & G. Marlatt (Eds.), *Addictive behaviors: Prevention and early intervention* (pp. 219–231). Amsterdam: Swets & Zeittinger.

Mosqueda, L. (1993). Assessment of rehabilitation potential. *Geriatric Rehabilitation, 9,* 689–700.

Neistadt, M. (1995). Methods of assessing client's priorities: A survey of adult physical dysfunction settings. *American Journal of Occupational Therapy, 49,* 428–436.

Nelson, D., & Stucky, C. (1992). The role of occupational therapy in preventing further disability of elderly persons in long-term care facilities. In J. Rothman & J. Levine (Eds.), *Prevention practice: Strategies for physical therapy and occupational therapy* (pp. 19–35). Philadelphia: Saunders.

Northen, J., Rust, D., Nelson, C., & Watts, J. (1995). Involvement of adult rehabilitation patients in setting occupational therapy goals. *American Journal of Occupational Therapy, 49,* 214–220.

Ornish, D. (1993). Changing life habits. In B. Moyers (Ed.), *The healing mind* (pp. 87–113). New York: Doubleday.

Peloquin, S. (1990). The patient–therapist relationship in occupational therapy: Understanding visions and images. *American Journal of Occupational Therapy, 44,* 13–21.

Rodin, J. (1986). Aging and health: Effects of the sense of control. *Science, 233,* 1271–1276.

Rogers, J. (1981). Gerontic occupational therapy. *American Journal of Occupational Therapy, 35,* 663–666.

Rogers, J. (1990). Improving the ability to perform daily tasks. In B. Kemp, K. Brunnell-Smith, & J. Ramsdell (Eds.), *Geriatric rehabilitation* (pp. 137–155). Boston: College-Hill Press.

Rosenfeld, M. (1984). Crisis intervention: The nuclear task approach. *American Journal of Occupational Therapy, 38,* 382–385.

Rosenfeld, M. (1990). A mid-career perspective of mental health practice. *Occupational Therapy in Mental Health, 12,* 47–61.

Rosenfeld, M. (1993). *Welles and lifestyle renewal: A manual for personal change.* Bethesda, MD: American Occupational Therapy Association.

Singer, I.B. (1953). The little shoemakers. In *Gimpel the fool.* New York: Fawcett Crest.

Slaikeu, K. (1984). *Crisis intervention: A handbook for practice and research.* Newton, MA: Allyn & Bacon.

Stevens-Ratchford, R. (1993). The effect of life review reminiscence activities on depression and self-esteem in older adults. *American Journal of Occupational Therapy, 47,* 413–420.

Strain, J., & Grossman, S. (1975). *Psychological care of the medically ill: A primer in liaison psychiatry.* New York: Appleton-Century-Crofts.

Taplin, J. (1971). Crisis theory: Critique and reformation. *Community Mental Health Journal, 7,* 13–23.

Van Etten, S. (1995). *Content validity of the measure of subacute rehabilitation potential.* Unpublished pilot study. Worcester, MA: Worcester State College.

Vargo, J. (1978). Some psychological effects of physical disabilities. *American Journal of Occupational Therapy, 32,* 1, 31–34.

Versluys, H. (1995). Evaluation of emotional adjustment to disabilities. In C. Trombly (Ed.), *Occupational therapy for physical dysfunction* (4th ed., pp. 225–234). Baltimore: Williams & Wilkins.

Victor, C. (1988). Approaches to the study of aging. In B. Gearing, M. Johnson, & T. Heller (Eds.), *Mental health problems in old age* (pp. 42–48). New York: Wiley.

Watson, L. (1986). Psychiatric consultation-liaison in the acute physical disabilities setting. *American Journal of Occupational Therapy, 40,* 338–342.

Watts, J., Kielhofner, G., Bauer, D., Gregory, M., & Valentine, D. (1986). The assessment of occupational functioning: A screening tool for use in long-term care. *American Journal of Occupational Therapy, 40,* 231–240.

Weintraub, R. (1995). *Psychiatric medicines in rehabilitation: What can they do?* Harvard Medical School Conference: Emotional Aspects of Physical Rehabilitation.

Zimmer-Branum, S., & Nelson, D. (1995). Occupationally embedded exercise versus rote exercise: A choice between occupational forms by elderly nursing home residents. *American Journal of Occupational Therapy, 49,* 397–402.

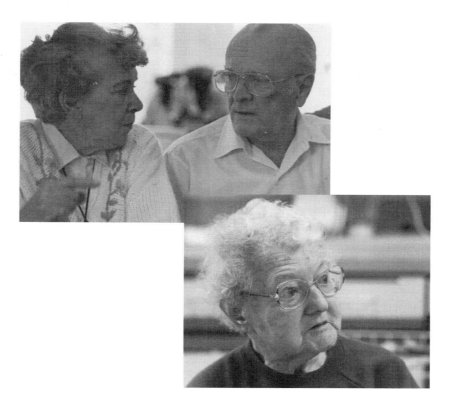

3

A Case Study Approach to Solving Complex Problems: Addressing Cognitive, Psychosocial, and Environmental Concerns

Susan E. Fasoli, MS, OTR/L

INTRODUCTION

The purpose of this chapter is to provide the reader with practical ideas that may be used to effectively treat individuals with challenging motivational issues. As we know, a holistic approach to occupational therapy intervention involves much more than increasing a patient's motion or improving a patient's ability to perform self-care. A brief discussion of environmental factors that influence how we provide services and an introduction to cognitive impairments precede the case studies. This information is intended to help the reader understand some of the variables that can affect an individual's needs and abilities and is summarized at the end of this chapter. The case studies that follow are accompanied by recommendations aimed at facilitating problem solving in similar therapeutic situations. Suggestions to help the reader best use these cases to enhance education or clinical practice may be found in this chapter as well.

The cases presented in this chapter represent the complexity of issues faced by occupational therapists. Demands placed on health care providers as a result of current reimbursement trends often lead to a concrete, function-oriented approach directed toward needs in self-care, functional mobility, or instrumental activities of daily living (IADL). The diminishing number of visits allowed for occupational therapy intervention also limits opportunities to establish therapeutic rapport with patients. This can affect the therapist's understanding of the complex emotional and life context issues that may be interfering with an individual's motivation for change. In developing a holistic approach to occupational therapy intervention, the therapist needs to explore life domains that are of importance to the individual receiving care, such as concerns with health maintenance, personal safety, psychological well-being and happiness, and free time usage (Clark et al., 1996). The practitioner must look beyond a patient's physical impairments and needs by actively engaging the individual in identifying his or her values, past and present interests, concerns, and desires. This approach involves the patient in the therapy program and assists with setting individualized goals for the future.

Occupational therapists must also consider the impact of environmental context and the availability of social support systems when working with an individual with motivational issues. Collaboration with the caregiver needs to occur whenever possible to maximize carryover of care and best identify not only the patient's needs but also the concerns of the caregiver. Clark, Corcoran, and Gitlin (1995) cited studies in which occupational therapists considered family members to be a barrier to effective treatment, particularly when the therapist's values for independence were not congruent with those of the caregiver. They also reported that caregivers' priorities involved the maintenance of routines and the assurance that no harm or loss of identity be experienced by the patient. Occupational therapists need to possess effective communication skills that will enable them to use open-ended questions to clearly identify needs and goals of the patient and family. Cultural background, previous routines and roles within the home and community, and ways in which the family has coped with adversity in the past must be explored. Although treatment sessions are limited by current reimbursement policies, the occupational therapist will be more effective in setting meaningful goals and establishing an effective treatment plan if time is taken to understand and clarify these complex psychosocial and environmental concerns early in the therapy program.

Occupational therapy education and procedures for evaluation in the clinic have traditionally focused on understanding and identifying deficiencies in occupational components, such as decreased sensation, strength, memory, or figure–ground skills. The assumption has been that these lower-level skills are prerequisite to the performance of occupational tasks, and that treatment of component skills will result in improved functional abilities (Trombly, 1995). Although it is now known that the practice of these component skills within the context of occupational tasks is needed for integration of learning to occur, many therapists continue to focus on the treatment of occupational components in isolation from occupational role performance. If we are to truly develop a holistic approach to intervention, occupational therapists must take a "top down" approach to evaluation by identifying occupational roles and tasks that the patient engaged in prior to treatment, and clarifying which tasks that individual will be responsible for when rehabilitation has ended (Trombly). If we then address deficient component skills within the context of important occupational roles and tasks, motivational obstacles should significantly decrease and treatment outcomes will be enhanced.

Some of the most frustrating cases encountered by therapists are often compounded by difficulty in distinguishing between cognitive deficits and motivational issues. An individual who has incurred frontal lobe damage and who presents with decreased initiation is often wrongly perceived as "unmotivated" by family members, who become frustrated by the patient's lack of participation in life roles and activities. Conversely, patients who have an awareness of their cognitive impairments may also display decreased motivation when they become depressed. The inability to perform occupational tasks, such as managing finances or reading a novel, because of difficulties with sustained attention, error recognition, or visual scanning can be discouraging and frustrating. Motivation and initiation are essential for effective and independent functioning. The occupational therapist needs to ask patients and families whether they have noted changes in these areas. The therapist should also observe the patient's behaviors and performance during meaningful tasks to determine if the individual is able to actively and spontaneously engage in activities that are interesting and motivating. If discrepancies are noted between these meaningful tasks and those considered more mundane by the patient (e.g., self-care, repetitive exercise programs), then motivational issues should be further investigated.

In their review of literature concerning changes in intelligence with normal aging, Bonder and Wagner (1994) reported that the most prominent age-related changes were apparent in the performance scale of the Wechsler Adult Intelligence Scale (WAIS and WAIS-Revised). Earlier and more significant declines were observed in measures of speed and accuracy in problem solving and in psychomotor and perceptual abilities. Vocabulary skill, general fund of information, and verbal comprehension and reasoning were not found to decline as individuals grew older.

Understanding the impact of normal aging on cognitive and perceptual abilities is important in enabling the occupational therapist to distinguish between behaviors that normally may be expected from those that indicate underlying neurological changes. The therapist needs to determine how cognitive and perceptual impairments may be contributing to altered occupational role performance and to intervene using either a remedial or adaptive approach.

A multitude of cognitive problems that may lead to motivational obstacles are identified in the complex cases that follow. One problem frequently cited in the case studies is impaired attention. The occupational therapist must examine the underlying behaviors that contribute to decreased attention to tasks. Does the patient appear to have a limited ability to shift attention between task components? Does he or she exhibit an inability to sustain or focus his or her attention, or conversely, does he or she display overattention to detail, interfering with attention to other task components? How much do the environmental or the task demands contribute to distractiblity? Does the patient attend better in a quiet environment? If the task demands are altered, does the patient's performance improve? An individual with attentional problems may benefit from working in a familiar, nondistracting environment with tasks that are meaningful. Observing task performance and questioning the patient about his or her approach to activities can provide the therapist with valuable information about underlying processing strategies and behaviors that interfere with attention and task completion (Toglia, 1993).

Memory impairments, particularly for immediate and delayed recall, are often observed when treating geriatric patients with neurological or psychiatric conditions. Deficits may be observed in declarative memory, such as the recall of facts or events, or in procedural memory, which includes memory for action, such as remembering how to operate a microwave oven (Toglia). Among the numerous factors that contribute to memory deficits are poor attention and organization of incoming information, which interfere with memory storage and retrieval. Memory deficits may affect all aspects of an individual's life, including role performance, maintenance of social relationships, and safety needs. An individual with memory deficits may become overly reliant on a structured routine and familiar environmental contexts in order to maintain functional abilities. Strategies such as training caregivers to provide consistent, repetitive, step-by-step cues or simple written directions for procedural learning may be helpful. Assisting the patient in associating new facts with something familiar and creating visual images of items to be remembered may facilitate attention, encoding, and subsequent recall (Toglia). Recognition cues such as "What vegetables do we need to buy at the store?" can help the individual with memory impairments to feel more capable in this area.

Difficulties with problem solving also are frequently observed in geriatric patients and are described in the case studies that follow. These difficulties may be caused by a number of variables, such as decreased speed of information processing, selection of inappropriate strategies, poor organization, or memory impairments (Bonder & Wagner, 1994). Problem-solving deficits can significantly affect an individual's ability to perform a wide range of familiar occupational tasks, such as finding a physician's telephone number in the telephone directory or driving an automobile. The occupational therapist can help to address these difficulties by observing the patient and asking him or her how he or she is planning to accomplish a particular activity. This information can help the therapist understand which cognitive elements may be deterring the patient's problem solving during occupational tasks. In addition, it is often beneficial to determine a patient's awareness of his or her capabilities and limitations by asking him or her to estimate or predict how well he or she will be able to perform functional activities. Individuals with decreased self-awareness will have difficulty anticipating and planning for potential problems and are at risk for developing safety concerns. The therapist may help the patient to better estimate performance demands through discussion and can help to organize information by breaking down tasks into smaller components. The therapist can assist with sequencing and memory by planning and by writing down steps needed to accomplish essential tasks. Again, the impact of environmental context on problem solving must be considered, and contextual cues should be used to enhance performance.

Ultimately, the therapist must remember that successful outcome of intervention is measured by enhanced ability to perform occupational roles and tasks rather than by improved memory or problem-solving abilities. The practitioner must plan treatment holistically and needs to recognize when remediation, adaptation, or compensation are most appropriate. Patients who have limited insight and are unable to judge their skills in relation to the demands of the task may benefit more from an adaptive functional approach in which therapy is geared toward educating the caregiver regarding the patient's limitations and identifying modifications that may enhance functional performance (Toglia, 1993).

The case of Mr. and Mrs. H. exemplifies many of the issues facing occupational therapists when working with elderly patients in the community. What follows is a recounting of the findings from their initial evaluations; a description of the support services they received; and the level of family involvement, analysis of the nuclear problem, and goals for intervention. Roles assumed by the occupational therapist and nuclear tasks incorporated in treatment are described.

CASE STUDY: MR. AND MRS. H.

Mr. and Mrs. H. were referred for occupational therapy services because of team concerns regarding their safety in remaining in their home environment. Mr. H. was a 77-year-old man diagnosed with Parkinson's disease 12 years prior to this referral, with a history of depression and benign tumors of the colon. During the initial evaluation session he was slow in responding to questions and benefited from step-by-step instructions and repetition for new learning. Although his sensation, range of motion (ROM), and strength in bilateral upper extremities were well within functional limits for his daily needs, his coordination was moderately slowed, with tremors and difficulty initiating movement noted at times. Mr. H.'s ambulation was characterized by a shuffling, often propulsive gait pattern, which contributed to occasional falls. Although he had walkers on both floors of his home, he tended to forget about them and relied on a straight cane during ambulation, much to his therapist's dismay. He often spent much of his time resting in bed and sleeping. His only occupation during the day was to search mortgagee foreclosure ads in the newspaper for his son's real estate business. He would often try to prepare breakfast for himself but would leave the kitchen in a state of disarray with burnt pans and spilled juice. He usually ate while standing at the counter to avoid the likelihood of dropping his plate as he carried it to the kitchen table 5 feet away. He relied on a home-health aide for self-care tasks, often not washing or dressing at all on days that the aide was not scheduled. His interactions with his wife of 52 years were limited to a few brief conversations a day. His goals for occupational therapy intervention were to be able to get around better and to do a little more for himself. However, he was resistant to change, stating that it was difficult for him to think about doing things differently or breaking away from the habits that provided continuity to his days. This appeared to be one way in which he was attempting to compensate for difficulties he was experiencing with memory.

Mrs. H., also 77 years old, was referred to occupational therapy following hospitalization to determine the cause of frequent falls. Her past medical history included cardiovascular disease, left lower extremity weakness secondary to polio as a child, and macular degeneration. Mrs. H. had been diagnosed as legally blind. During the initial evaluation, she was able to clearly communicate her needs but demonstrated decreased safety awareness during ambulation. She was able to walk around her home with the use of a straight cane while reaching for walls or furniture with her other hand to ensure balance. Her upper extremity sensation, ROM, and strength were essentially within functional limits for daily needs. Her coordination, however, was impaired for tasks such as handwriting because of her visual deficits and mild tremors in her hands. She managed sponge bathing and dressing without assistance, and did what she could to wash dishes and pick up the kitchen. Mrs. H. spent much of the day listening to talk radio while sitting on her bed in her own room. She related that she used to enjoy cooking and knitting but had not performed these activities to any extent since her vision had declined. Her goals for therapy were to be able to do things better in spite of her poor vision.

Mr. and Mrs. H. were fortunate in that they were receiving support from a variety of community and state agencies. They both received occupational and physical therapies and nursing services from the local Visiting Nurse Association (VNA). Mr. H. had home-health aide assistance 3–4 times a week. Meals on Wheels provided both lunch and dinner 5 days weekly. Mrs. H. was peripherally followed by the Commission for the Blind, but services and training in the use of visual aides were quite limited. Their insurance company was a health maintenance organization (HMO), and their caseworker attempted to provide necessary services within the financial constraints placed upon her. However, a total of only six occupational therapy visits was allowed for both Mr. and Mrs. H to address their complex issues. The community nurse from their town helped them gain access to an emergency call system. She also provided a machine on a trial basis that dispensed medications to Mr. H. in a timely fashion, in an attempt to avoid missed doses (which happened frequently). Their son had hired a homemaker who cleaned and did laundry once a week. In spite of these interventions, their home was constantly in a state of disarray and badly in need of painting and cleaning. In fact, during the treatment program the kitchen was totally remodeled, a process that posed significant safety issues for several weeks. The patients' only son was very busy with his real estate business and was extremely difficult to contact to discuss his parents' needs. Recommendations to repair and add railings to indoor and outdoor stairways and to improve lighting within the home went unheeded. Although the son was available to take his parents to physician's appointments, his involvement with them was quite limited. Luckily, Mr. and Mrs. H. could call on their elderly next-door neighbor as needed to manage the trash or shut off the stove when they could not figure out how to use their new range. Obviously, the support that these individuals received from outside services was essential in maintaining their precarious living situation. They were both strongly opposed to alternate living situations such as retirement communities or long-term-care placements. Great effort was made to keep communication as open as possible among these varied team members.

Although the initial evaluation assessed occupational component skills such as motor abilities and cognition, the nuclear problem addressed in treatment focused on overcoming threats to Mr. and Mrs. H.'s safety and level of independence, thereby enabling them to continue to reside in their own home for as long as possible. Generally, occupational therapy goals for both Mr. and Mrs. H. were to enhance safe functional mobility and transfers within the home, to enhance self-care abilities, and to provide training and visual aids to improve safety in the home, particularly in the kitchen. Further recommendations for installation of equipment such as a long-handled hose in the shower were made to their son with some success. Nuclear tasks were identified with Mr. and Mrs. H. to help them sustain occupational patterns such as simple breakfast preparation and to learn new vital skills. Simple directions were writ-

ten for Mr. H. to facilitate the procedural memory needed to recall how to operated the microwave, and large visual aids were applied to the stove in an attempt to teach both Mr. and Mrs. H. safe operation of the stove top. Repetitive problem-solving scenarios were presented to Mrs. H. to help her plan how to most effectively use their new emergency call system in the case of an accident, knowing that the couple occasionally forgot the call button in the bathroom after bathing or left it on the bedside table. The occupational therapist spent time removing the old toilet seat so the commode would properly fit over the toilet and adapted the height of chairs to enable Mr. H. to safely rise to standing. These tasks were remotivating to Mr. H. in that they demonstrated that he could get around the house more safely and easily. Lighting in the home was improved by opening drapes that had been closed for years and by adding light bulbs to ceiling fixtures. Time was also spent with Mrs. H. reorganizing drawers and cabinets in the new kitchen to help her locate needed items, as well as to discard unnecessary kitchen supplies. During the treatment sessions, time was allotted to discuss how Mr. and Mrs. H. were coping with their limitations, how they might be most satisfied with their life situation, and what they desired for the future. These discussions reopened communication between spouses as well. Despite the limited number of occupational therapy sessions they received because of funding restrictions, these individuals were able to develop a relationship with the occupational therapist, which helped motivate them to undertake change and attempt to take back some degree of control in their lives.

The level of success achieved in treating Mr. and Mrs. H. can be partially attributed to an effort to provide adaptations within the context of their daily routine in their home environment. It was necessary to respect their need for consistency to partially compensate for the cognitive challenges they were experiencing. The occupational therapist had to put aside her own values and ideals for an optimal situation and learned a lot about their perceived needs by asking open-ended questions and clarifying what they said to ensure understanding. Fortunately, during this short intervention phase, some strategies and adaptations were made to enhance Mr. and Mrs. H.'s safety and ability to remain in their home. However, ongoing reevaluation will be needed to identify how to best accommodate their changing needs.

◆   ◆   ◆

The following cases have been included because they describe challenging motivational issues faced in a variety of clinical settings with a wide range of diagnoses. Some of the case studies have been presented by the treating occupational therapist and responded to by experienced clinicians. Others have been written entirely by the occupational therapist providing intervention to identify techniques that were most effective in facilitating participation and motivation. It is important to remember that the responses to these situations provide one approach to

intervention and are not necessarily the *only* correct approach.

Before reading the cases it may be helpful to review the theoretical concepts and definitions in chapter 2. The following questions may be used to apply these concepts to the case studies and to develop your own clinical reasoning skills. Try to answer these questions yourself prior to reading the responses that follow each case. Also, determine what additional information may be needed to develop an effective therapeutic approach.

◆ Determine the *nuclear problem* by (a) identifying the precipitating event and (b) discovering the meaning of this event and the resulting impairment or disability to the patient.

◆ What *resources* are available to help in this situation, e.g., what level of participation are the individual's coping history, social supports, and current level of effort?

◆ What *stage of response* to this injury or illness is the patient in? Is this patient in shock, acknowledgment, or adjustment? How might this stage influence his or her motivation toward rehabilitation?

◆ What is the *goal* of motivational intervention? What do the patient and therapist hope to achieve?

◆ What *therapeutic approach* do you think will be most effective? Is it best to provide affective management and support, or to focus on cognitive restoration? What degree of challenge is the patient ready to accept?

- What *nuclear tasks* would be most beneficial in addressing the nuclear problem? What types of tasks (expressive activities, functional skills, remotivating activities, and so forth) may be most effective?

In addition, you may choose to evaluate the patient's rehabilitation potential by using the Measure of Subacute Rehabilitation Potential described in chapter 12. You might also apply Kemp's equation, as described in chapter 2, to determine the individual's motivation for rehabilitation.

Whenever possible, try to make this learning process as interactional as possible by discussing your responses with fellow students or clinicians. It is hoped that this experience will further develop your clinical reasoning skills and enhance your effectiveness when treating individuals with motivational issues in the clinic.

KEY POINTS

- The practitioner must look beyond a patient's physical impairments and needs by actively engaging the individual in identifying his or her values, past and present interests, and concerns and desires.

- Occupational therapists must also consider the effect of environmental context and the availability of social support systems when investigating needs and goals of the patient and family.

- The practice of occupational components, such as decreased sensation, strength, memory, or figure–ground skills, needs to occur within the context of occupational tasks in order for integration of learning to occur.

- An individual who has incurred frontal lobe damage and who presents with decreased initiation is often wrongly perceived as "unmotivated" by family members.

- The most prominent age-related changes in normal individuals are apparent in the performance scale of the Wechsler Adult Intelligence Scale (WAIS and WAIS-Revised): vocabulary skills, general fund of information, and verbal comprehension and reasoning have not been found to decline significantly as individuals age.

- An individual with attentional problems may benefit from working in a familiar, nondistracting environment with tasks that are meaningful.

- Observing task performance and questioning the patient about his or her approach to activities can provide the therapist with valuable information about underlying processing strategies and behaviors that interfere with attention and task completion (e.g., limited ability to shift attention, overattention to detail, and so forth).

- Memory impairments may be observed in declarative memory, such as the recall of facts or events, or in procedural memory, which includes memory for action, such as remembering how to operate a microwave oven. Strategies may include use of consistent, repetitive, step-by-step cues or simple written directions for procedural learning. Creating visual images of items to be remembered may facilitate attention, encoding, and subsequent recall. Recognition cues can help the individual with memory impairments to feel more capable in this area.

◆ Difficulties with problem solving may be caused by a number of variables, such as decreased speed of information processing, selection of inappropriate strategies, poor organization, or memory impairments. The therapist may help the patient to organize information by breaking down tasks into smaller components. He or she can assist with sequencing and memory by planning and by writing down steps needed to accomplish essential tasks.

◆ Individuals with decreased self-awareness will have difficulty anticipating and planning for potential problems and are at risk for developing safety concerns.

◆ The practitioner must plan treatment holistically and needs to recognize when remediation, adaptation, or compensation are most appropriate.

REFERENCES

Bonder, B.R., & Wagner, M.B. (1994). *Functional performance in older adults.* Philadelphia: F.A. Davis.

Clark, C.A., Corcoran, M., & Gitlin, L.N. (1995). An exploratory study of how occupational therapists develop therapeutic relationships with family caregivers. *American Journal of Occupational Therapy, 49,* 587–594.

Clark, F., Carlson, M., Zemke, R., Frank, G., Patterson, K., Ennevor, B.L., Rankin-Martinez, A., Hobson, L., Crandal, J., Mandel, D., & Lipson, L. (1996). Life domains and adaptive strategies of a group of low-income well older adults. *American Journal of Occupational Therapy, 50,* 99–108.

Toglia, J. (1993). Attention and memory. In C.B. Royeen (Ed.), *AOTA self study series: Cognitive rehabilitation* (lesson 4). Bethesda, MD: American Occupational Therapy Association.

Trombly, C.A. (ed.). (1995). *Occupational therapy for physical dysfunction* (4th ed.). Baltimore: Williams & Wilkins.

Case Studies

A PATIENT PUNISHES THE STAFF

The patient is a 71-year-old female who was born in New Bedford to Greek-speaking parents. She had three siblings and she was the second oldest child. According to the patient, her family was very strict and physically abusive. Greek was spoken at home. The patient had no formal education and was not allowed to have friends or even date. At 19 years of age, the patient met her husband. They had two children. According to the patient, her husband was aggressive. They subsequently divorced. The patient's daughter is a drug addict and is estranged from the patient. Her son was shot to death 11 years ago during a criminal interaction in the city. The patient took in her grandson and brought him up on her own. The patient worked as a housekeeper and also received a diploma in seamstressing, of which she is very proud.

The patient was living alone in a first-floor apartment of housing for the elderly, receiving daily home-health aid to assist her with a.m. and p.m. care, and homemaking services with a visiting nurse at least once a week. Meals on Wheels was also received. The patient was seen on an outpatient basis at regular times for long-standing depression.

The patient sustained an oblique fracture mid-shaft to the right femur with posterior displacement of distal fracture. The patient was admitted to the skilled nursing facility 2 ½ weeks later to receive rehabilitation after undergoing an open reduction of internal fragments to the right femur. Past medical history includes recurrent major depression, sciatic palsy to the right leg with footdrop since a total hip replacement in 1991. She also had back surgery three times. Other diagnoses include moderate dementia, hypertension, cellulitis of the right foot, myxedema, and urinary tract infection.

During her stay at the skilled nursing facility, the patient received occupational and physical therapy services on three different occasions following fluctuations and changes in the patient's medical and psychiatric status. Five months after admission to the skilled nursing facility, the patient was admitted to the psychiatric unit at the hospital after becoming increasingly upset, angry, and lashing out at the caregivers. Prior to her hospitalization, the patient became temperamental, was unable to sleep, and refused her meals and medication. She stated that she was trying to punish the staff. The patient returned to the skilled nursing facility after 1 week of treatment and being placed on the following medications: Zoloft, Valium, Haldol, Zantac, and Desyrel. The patient was placed in a double room farther away from the nurses' desk. She also did not tolerate roommates.

The patient's way of dealing with disappointment is by getting angry, verbally lashing out at persons around her, and refusing her treatment or care.

The patient loves her grandson but every time she sees or speaks to him, she gets upset and blames her grandson's girlfriend for taking him away from her. The patient carries her cigarettes, lighter, gum, and photographs of herself from about 25–30 years ago in her pocketbook at all times. She believes that when she goes home, she will be able to regain her figure as in the photos and walk in high heels again.

She does not trust anyone easily, especially after she was told by her visiting nurse that she would only stay at the facility for 2 weeks.

The patient's Greek culture and beliefs are important to her and this comes across in her actions. She gets very upset and angry about her long stay at the facility and not being able to return home or to visit her parents' and son's graves on religious holidays.

The patient requires minimal assistance with grooming and upper body dressing; moderate assistance with bathing, bed mobility, and toileting; maximal assistance with her lower body dressing, bed to wheelchair transfers, and homemaking skills. Her identified impairments include impaired physical endurance, learning and memory limitations, impaired attention and concentration span, poor safety awareness, generalized weakness, limited ROM of right lower extremity, poor dynamic sitting and standing balance, localized pain, and depression. The patient has a long leg brace for her right leg, uses a standard walker, and presently walks with the rehabilitation aide.

Occupational therapy goals are for the patient to attain her optimal level of independence with self-care and transfers. Treatment plan includes skilled occupational therapy service six times a week for 4 weeks for ADL self-care; and residential ADL training with functional endurance, transfer, balance, and safety awareness training. Education for the patient, staff, and family is required regarding the patient's functional capabilities and for cognitive training with respect to reality orientation, insight, problem solving, and appropriate communication style and techniques.

The patient is cooperative in her therapy when she is able to smoke outside at appointed times during the day after her treatment sessions.

The therapist's problem or dilemma is mainly that the patient becomes extremely upset, angry, and resistive when asked to perform her exercise or self-care tasks. Various home-health agencies have screened the patient and not accepted her for home care by withdrawing their services. The patient presently remains at the facility. The patient continuously threatens to go home by cab against her doctor's orders. She does not realize that she would be on her own at home without community services if she signs herself out. She demonstrates impaired insight and knowledge regarding her own capabilities and limitations.

—*Ute Gruner, OTR/L*

Answer

Psychosocial dysfunction is a major obstacle to rehabilitation in this case. Due to a life history of deprivation and abuse, this individual does not have the emotional resources to cope with disability or with treatment. She may realistically fear becoming a permanent resident of the facility and losing her home. Her petulant behavior in response to crisis probably will cause her therapists to feel helpless and angry. When patients are persistantly resistant and abusive, early discharge from occupational therapy services is a likely result.

Several psychosocial factors should be considered. This patient experienced abuse at an early age at the hands of primary caretakers. She was prevented from making supportive friendships. Because of trauma suffered when she was young and emotionally vulnerable, she has not learned to cope with the stresses of life. Sadly, her life has involved a long series of such stresses: abuse from her husband, traumatic death of her son, alienation from her daughter, and a sequence of serious illnesses, injuries, and surgery. Given her history, illness and pain may seem like familiar punishments to her. In pain, she regresses to an infantile level. Lacking any substantial nurturing experience, she never established basic trust with others and cannot readily accept nurturance or support. Left only with her feelings of frustration, helplessness and anger, she spills them into the environment, pulling her therapists into her emotional experience. Her hostile, irrational behavior causes others (home-health providers, for example) to reject her, ironically replicating the rejection and abandonment she has already suffered. Her statement about the girl-friend taking her grandson from her is a clear expression of her stance in life as an unfairly abused and abandoned child.

Several positive factors noted include significant relationships and accomplishments. The patient's pride in completing a seamstress course, working as a housekeeper, and raising her grandson represent positive elements in her life history. She has risen above adversity in at least three areas and has completed important tasks. Also, the patient may have sustained a long-term connection with a psychotherapist, given her years of treatment for depression. This relationship should be investigated and rekindled if possible, or a new therapist found to address her psychosocial needs. Her relationship with her grandson is of tremendous importance, and regular contact with him should be strongly encouraged by the staff.

But how can we treat such an irrational and irascible patient? How do we establish trust and common ground? Limit setting, consistency, straight talk, occupational engagement, and collaboration are the central tenets of an effective approach.

Limit setting: Tell the patient you cannot permit her to be abusive and punishing to you and others. Remind her that she knows how terrible abuse can be from her own experience. She does not want to be the cause of that kind of pain, does she? Tell her you will end contact whenever she is verbally abusive and not return until the next day. But also encourage her to put her feelings into words so that you can help her with her pain and troubles. Congratulate her when she does so appropriately.

Consistency: Show up every day at an established time. Do exactly what you have said you will do. Build trust by being consistent, unflappable, and respectful. Never rise to the bait or act in an angry way with this patient, and you will have a chance to help her grow.

She will learn to contain her emotions from your healthy modelling.

Straight talk: Tell her she has been very sick, that she will need a lot of care and treatment to improve enough to return home or even to enjoy life at the facility. Insist that she will ruin her chances if she pushes her helpers away. Put the choice about treatment involvement in her hands (it is, you know). Create a tracking form to hang on her wall, so you can recognize the number of sessions completed and the goals achieved as you go along. Whenever the patient creates obstacles to treatment, stop the action and confront the obstacle.

Occupational engagement: Housekeeping, seamstressing, and her appearance are interests that can be meaningfully and productively pursued in occupational therapy sessions. The patient possessed professional housekeeping skills in younger days. She will need to use these skills after returning home. Go with her strength. Let her instruct you in the kitchen or in straightening her room. Sew a simple project together. Again, let her take the lead. This occupation may be comforting while also benefitting cognitive and fine motor performance. Finally, take a look at that picture of the patient in her twenties. How can she restore her appearance now? Washing and setting her hair, doing her nails and makeup are elements of ADL with which to begin. She will never be 25 again, but she can look her best. Get her to tell you about herself in those days. She remembers herself positively in that part of her life.

Collaboration: This patient's life and her medical condition have gotten seriously out of control. Help her regain a sense of control. Give her choices at every turn. Be her partner whenever possible. Believe in her ability to make good choices and to mobilize her strengths. Most important, accept her sensible goals for treatment and put them first on your list. Once you have helped her to do something important to her, even something small, she will be more ready to follow your lead.

Finally, if treatment is highly successful, advocacy and a great deal of care must be devoted to transitional discharge plans and relationship building with community caregivers. There are some fences to mend. Given the patient's cognitive deficits and thin social supports, a gradual transition to life in the facility is a more likely outcome.

The treatment approach described above requires a great deal of the treatment team. However, that is frequently the case when patients have multiple and serious physical, cognitive and psychosocial problems. Sometimes even Herculean efforts are unsuccessful. But in other instances, the therapist who struggles to find a way, brings a person back from the edge of the abyss.

—*Mark S. Rosenfeld, PhD, OTR/L*

◆   ◆   ◆

OVERCOMING DEPENDENCY AND INFANTILIZATION

Mr. W., a 70-year-old, married male came to our rehabilitation hospital with a history of right cerebrovascular accident (CVA) with left-sided hemiplegia. He had the CVA a year prior to actually coming to rehabilitation and at that time had been placed in a nursing home, having been told that he would be dependent on others from this point on. Prior to his CVA, Mr. W. had been living an independent, active lifestyle and was now having tremendous difficulty adapting to his current limitations. Mr. W.'s lifestyle previously emphasized involvement with crafts and with intellectual pursuits. Mr. W. was a retired upholsterer and continued to enjoy doing light handiwork around the home. Mr. W. liked to keep his hands busy and was often involved in some type of craftsmanship. Mr. W. also enjoyed engaging in cultural activities with his wife; living just outside Manhattan provided them with the opportunity for frequent trips to museums and the theater.

Mr. W.'s wife was extremely supportive, perhaps a bit overinvolved, taking away from Mr. W.'s real need to care for himself or be assertive about his treatment regimen.

Mr. W. came to us wheelchair dependent, unable to dress or bathe himself, and unable to move from bed to chair. His goal was to gain enough function to enable him to return to his home and spend several hours alone during the day while his wife worked. He was emotionally invested in this goal, but allowed himself to fall into the "sick role," believing that as long as he was in the hospital others would care for him. Mr. W. coped with the decrease in his health by withdrawing into himself and relinquishing control to others.

Occupational therapy goals for Mr. W. included gaining greater independence in dressing skills, bed mobility,

and transfers. Mr. W. was scheduled to be seen daily by occupational therapy for 45–90 minutes each day. The treatment plan included a daily ADL program, as well as training in the various component skills needed to transfer successfully. This included a combination of mat activities, as well as actual transfer practice to a variety of surfaces.

Although Mr. W. stated that he was in agreement with the treatment plan and goals, he had difficulty gathering up the motivation to physically participate. During treatment times, Mr. W. complained of headaches, stomachaches, and severe fatigue. Mr. W. would act almost childlike in his excuses to leave treatment sessions early. Mr. W. appeared truly overwhelmed by the enormity of his situation and lacked the motivation to help himself look past his current status and forward toward the progress that the future could bring.

The occupational therapist's problem in this case was how to help motivate this patient, who clearly had the ability to make progress. This patient appeared to possess the necessary movement and physical capabilities to make gains in occupational therapy if there was a way to help him become more invested in his occupational therapy program.

—*Karen Halfon, OTR/L*

Answer

It seems that the nuclear problem for Mr. W. is his sudden and complete removal physically and emotionally from his life tasks, i.e., his role of retired craftsman who enjoys working with his hands and his avocational pursuit of cultural activities in the Manhattan area. How or why he was relocated to the Boston area was not shared; however, the fact that he is now here tells the therapist that he has suffered from two episodes of "catastrophic relocation"—the first being to a nursing home following the acute insult with a very discouraging prognosis, and the second being that he is not being "rehabilitated" in his familiar Manhattan environment. Despite the fact that the wife is described as extremely supportive, the support is extended in such a way that infantilizes him, perhaps out of guilt or feelings of helplessness on her part as she deals with the changing roles within her family unit. Nonetheless, the losses that the patient has experienced block his participation as long as the "rehabilitation process" is *applied to* him rather than *in collaboration with* him.

To attend to routine ADL retraining without exploring the importance of these tasks with Mr. W. sets both the patient and the therapist up for a frustrating experience. Nursing home life has already taught him that these basic needs will be taken care of for him, regardless of how childlike his behavior becomes. No one stays naked or unfed for long. Help will be provided, solicited or not. If the tasks can be related to the recovery of one of his losses, then engagement in the retraining should be easier. If, for example, donning a smock coverall type shirt would protect his regular clothing from stain splatters or sawdust, then this task has a meaning other than basic upper body dressing. Cleaning of a paint brush or vacuuming sawdust has the elements of basic home

management. A trip to a local Boston, while not Manhattan, museum with the therapist may give a reason to select an outfit other than a pull-on jogging suit to wear—hence, lower body dressing, community mobility, and avocational time use. Enlisting the expertise of this craftsman as a consultant to a project the therapist is planning might be a basic bridge that spans the sense of loss. The sharing of past successes through photographs of past projects Mr. W. has completed, or reminiscence-oriented experiences, can reinforce that he has an adult skill to give in exchange for the "childlike" skill set he needs to reacquire. All of "the necessary movement" in the world will not open the door if the individual possessing that movement can see no functional purpose to raising his hand to the door knob.

I would capitalize upon these first small success steps to develop a realistic treatment plan *with* Mr. W. based upon *listening* to him to learn very specifically what is important to him. Therapists often feel the need to "fill in the silence" too quickly, rather than to allow patients adequate time to formulate their thoughts and wishes and share them. Be patient with your patient! Remember that the basic tenet of occupational therapy is Ability through Activity—not through mat activities, pegs, and cones, but by engaging the patient in an activity upon which *he* or *she* has placed meaning toward achieving *his* or *her* goals, regardless of where these goals fit in the official medical treatment plan's priority list. Through active, focused listening and individualized planning, the barriers to independence can be reduced as specific functional behaviors, which have generalized application, are acquired. Any activity should be considered therapeutic because all tasks are really a component of an activity of daily living. The successful therapist works *with* the patient to select tasks that meet the specific need and build toward the mutually desired goals.

—*Gail Wolfe, MBA, OTR/L*

◆　　◆　　◆

NO TREATMENT NEEDED— GO HOME OR BUST!

Mary S. is a 66-year-old, divorced female admitted with a primary diagnosis of CABG, peripheral neuropathy, and a previous CVA with residual weakness. Mary lived alone prior to coming into the hospital and, per patient report, "was functionally independent." The patient has one son who lives across the country and has contact with his mother only by telephone calls.

Mary retired a few years ago from her position as a clerk in a small business. She has not supplemented her free time with any new avocations. She continues to enjoy doing crossword puzzles and watching television. She has a few friends who visit her, but she seldom leaves her home.

The thought of being in the hospital is very difficult for Mary to deal with. Despite the fact that she has difficulty bathing, dressing, ambulating, transferring, and completing most activities of daily living, Mary is quite resistant to therapy. Mary believes that the only means for getting better is to go home.

She would be able to handle everything if she went home. Unfortunately, this is far from the truth.

The goals established for Mary (she refused to participate in goal setting) in occupational therapy are realistic— home with some assistance. Mary will not participate in any therapies, however, stating she does not need them. The son is threatening to put his mother in a nursing home. It became very difficult to justify having the patient in a rehabilitation hospital.

It was increasingly difficult to motivate Mary or even to speak to her. She did not appear depressed, just adamant in her decisions. Mary became hostile to staff. The dilemma for the staff became whether to continue to try to involve the patient in therapy to achieve her one long-term goal of going home while being sometimes verbally abused by the patient. The other option was to leave the patient alone and allow the patient to be discharged to a nursing home.

—*Kelley Drane Fleming, OTR/L*

Answer

To analyze Mary S.'s nuclear problem, initially one would have to address the issue of goal setting. The therapist states that Mary refused to participate in goal setting, yet Mary has made her objective clear, and that is to return home, the only place where she can recover. This is certainly not an uncommon set of circumstances: an independent elder, comfortable with a fairly solitary lifestyle, who resists the intrusion of the hectic rehabilitation hospital setting and demands to go home, seemingly oblivious to the safety concerns of others. By her own report, Mary was "functionally independent" before admission and apparently sees no obstacle to returning to the same level. The discrepancy between Mary's and the therapist's views of expected level of functioning may be due to a number of factors: denial, a difference in standard, or perhaps poor judgment related to cognitive deficits. Presuming that Mary's mental status would indeed allow her to comprehend the risks involved in independent living, then a closer look at Mary's previous coping skills would be indicated. Previous to retirement, Mary's life may have centered on her worker role. She has few friends who visit her, but she did not venture out to discover new friends once her job ceased to provide her with consistent socialization. Her "adaptation" to increased free time was a continuation of old favorite pastimes, which also were solitary and sedentary. Change is difficult for her and family supports appear limited at best. As the environment becomes more confrontational, Mary digs in her heels and becomes abusive, resisting attempts to reality test her perceptions, and allowing her to reinforce her denial of the gravity of the present circumstances.

Recognition of her needs for privacy and independence would be initial treatment steps, cradled in an atmosphere that brought control back to the patient. (Why is it that her son can determine her discharge to a nursing home?). Home provides familiar surroundings, structure, and freedom from intrusion. Would Mary help us create a facsimile for her stay in the rehabilitation setting?

Since she valued her worker role previously, would she accept this recovery period as her contribution to a productive lifestyle, her "job" being to learn a new way to transfer and ambulate safely? Once the therapist identifies necessary steps leading to discharge, Mary needs to prioritize, expressing what tasks she feels are most important for her to do independently and which she can accept assistance with; which tasks mean the most to her and which she could delay until discharge to home care. The staff must admit that some goals can be better met at home and accept Mary's view that she can regain sustaining abilities more easily in her own place and in her own way.

—Jacqueline R. Brennan, RPT/L,
MS, OTR/L

◆   ◆   ◆

CVA IN SURGERY: CAN HE BOUNCE BACK?

Mr. Y. is a 67-year-old, semiretired, never married male of Scandinavian descent who suffered a right CVA during a CABG 1 month ago. He has a history of hypertension and arthritis in the left shoulder. At the initial interview the should pain was "tolerable." Passive range of motion (ROM) was intact on the left without flexion synergy. He has some active motion in all joints of the arm and hand. Sensation is intact.

Mr. Y. received intensive rehabilitation in a center for 3 weeks and will be followed by an occupational therapist in his one-bedroom apartment 1–3 times per week. Originally from Minnesota, he has lived in New York City for 30 years. He has no living relatives but has many male friends who call and visit.

Mr. Y. was a tenured professor of political science with an expertise in Latin America. His hobbies are playing the piano and bookbinding. He is also interested in furniture and artifacts.

Mr. Y. is depressed, angry, anxious, and expresses angst and concern over his plight. He claims that he never was tough and feels he is starting to fall apart, cannot concentrate, and feels "wobbly."

Occupational therapy short-term goals are to increase strength and ROM in the left upper extremity, to decrease pain in left shoulder, and to prepare a cold meal. Long-term goals are for the left upper extremity to be a good functional assist and for Mr. Y. to manage his own shoulder pain and be independent in meal preparation.

Mr. Y.'s depression and anger are motivational issues. He spends sessions complaining about his bad luck and forgets (or does not follow) his home exercise plan.

—Jane Sorensen, PhD, OTR/L

Answer

Mr. Y. went into surgery expecting to come out "healed"; instead, he came out "crippled."

The first occupational therapy goal should be to alleviate depression. I feel that by relieving his depression, the anger and lack of concentration will diminish. The description of his disability does not indicate cognitive damage, which is a major interfering factor with rehabilitation success.

I would not try any physical interventions for a few sessions. I would just talk with him. What was he hoping to do after his surgery? How did he like teaching? What did he teach? Ask him about interesting art or craft pieces in his apartment. Culturally, Scandinavians honor stoicism. By allowing and encouraging discussion, you will give him a chance to regain his composure.

I would introduce "faux stained glass" (Sun Catchers) as an activity to use his left hand as a good assist. The bright color will further alleviate his depression. The design should complement his decor. This activity also provides a successful experience within his new physical reality and is emotionally stabilizing.

Once Mr. Y. is engaged in the stained glass activity, introduce his home exercise program (HEP). Explain exactly what the exercise will do to his physiology. Remember, you are dealing with an intellectual, so you will get a better response when you engage his mind.

Mr. Y.'s prognosis is good for occupational therapy. He probably will never regain full function of his arm, but he should be able to resume his life with vigor and satisfaction.

—Jane Sorensen, PhD, OTR

◆   ◆   ◆

A PARTNERSHIP OF FUN AND ACCOMPLISHMENT

Sally B. was referred for occupational therapy services in her home following a short hospital stay because of complications of postpolio syndrome. She is a

74-year-old woman, who had, in addition to her presenting diagnosis, a history of mild mental retardation and speech difficulties. She had been cared for by her mother and other relatives in the past but now relies on assistance by hired caregivers for both personal care and housekeeping tasks. Before the recent exacerbation of the polio symptoms, she had been able to assist with or independently perform simple dressing and grooming tasks and was mobile within her small home using a light, manual wheelchair. Her current difficulties include a decreased use of her dominant right upper extremity and lowered respiratory endurance. Oral-motor skills are also affected and a gastrostomy tube has been inserted to ensure proper nutrition without risk of aspiration.

Even with her physical disabilities, Sally has always sought to be as independent as possible, both in her personal care and during outside-the-home activities. Born well before the current time when handicapped persons are more integrated into society, Sally's family made efforts to provide her with community activities and she served as a volunteer in situations such as the local library. As her physical abilities lessened, i.e., moving from forearm crutches to reliance on wheelchair transport, she has become more isolated and dependent on others for travel outside the home. She is very motivated to regain her prehospitalization level of ability, as she does not want to be any more dependent on others than she already is.

Because of her supportive care regarding ADL, Sally and the occupa-

tional therapist planned to initially concentrate on regaining physical abilities (active ROM, strength, endurance over her right upper extremity, and improvement of respiratory endurance for all tasks) before formulating compensatory strategies. Oral-motor retraining was also addressed to prepare for removal of the gastrostomy tube. Therapy frequency was two to three sessions per week, with the caregiver present to ensure more carryover regarding strategies and exercise programs.

In addition to the physical rehabilitation concerns, the therapist also has to take into account Sally's motivational obstacles of cognitive delays in formulating treatment activities. Working with developmentally disabled adults always presents a challenge because typical teaching methods may not be effective. Many patients may not have an internal motivation to improve their skills, and instead may respond to treatment activities with "if it's not fun, I'm not going to do it!" In Sally's case, she is motivated to improve, but her attention span is shorter than usual and she tires of activities quickly. In devising specific activities to address her rehabilitation needs, the therapist mentions that a good activity to improve upper extremity mobility and respiratory endurance is blowing bubbles using a wand. Sally becomes excited and shares that she has never had the opportunity to blow bubbles and insists that this activity be included in the plan. During subsequent sessions, she appears to thoroughly enjoy the time spent with the bubble wand and makes good progress in regaining physical and respiratory skills, with improvements also seen in time on task behaviors.

The therapist's dilemma is to develop therapy approaches and activities that resolve concerns while engaging the patient in the process. This is an ongoing challenge for any therapist. In this case, the patient also has the complications of cognitive delays and speech concerns that could be an obstacle to treatment planning.

—*Dawn Morrill, MS, OTR*

Answer

The nuclear problem for Sally B. is the continuing decline in independence due to her medical diagnosis and preexisting conditions. Sally's independence is important to her because she does not want to depend on others for assistance, but due to deteriorating abilities, she has become dependent for travel.

Sally is internally motivated but has a decreased attention span, so activities must be short, interesting, and provide a positive outcome (i.e., blowing bubbles). She has past experience in volunteering and participating in community activities. A new volunteer activity may include a nursing home setting where Sally delivers the mail, which is color coded with stickers, to each room or resident. Occupational therapy treatment goals for physical abilities would be met (i.e., Sally would deliver mail with her dominant hand in her wheelchair so goals of active ROM, strength, and respiratory endurance could improve) and since each resident or room would be "new" or "different," Sally may remain interested. The number of residents or rooms could fluctuate according to Sally's attention span. Residents love to receive mail and Sally would benefit from their positive attitude toward seeing her.

Sally's ability to help others may provide her with a feeling of accomplishment that she can help others. If Sally's medical condition deteriorates gradually over time, she may accept that she needs help but is still able to help others. The mail task can be modified as her medical status changes.

—*Joanne M. Gallagher, MS, OTR/L*

❖   ❖   ❖

TOO MUCH PAIN FOR THE COMEBACK KID?

Mrs. X. is a 65-year-old, married woman with six children, admitted to a subacute rehabilitation center with the diagnosis of a total left knee replacement. The replacement was performed as a result of arthritis of many years' duration. Prior to admission, she had been living at home with her second husband. All six children are grown and married; three are very supportive. She has several grandchildren and one great-grandchild. Her vocation has been as a certified nursing assistant while rearing her children. She "had to work" because her first husband abandoned her and the children. She had always enjoyed knitting and parlayed this talent into a custom blanket and sweater business, which she did part time. Her current husband of 5 years is a retired custodial engineer; she has been retired for about 10 years. They enjoy a mutual interest in gourmet cooking shows and often experiment together at mealtimes. Their network of friends encompasses a wide variety of new and old acquaintances. While a resident, she made and received a multitude of telephone calls daily from family and friends.

The patient's goal is to exit the rehabilitation center as soon as possible so that "someone else who really needs the bed" can use it. However, she realizes her rehabilitation is essential and timely for return home. In an interview, she divulges that she had an auto accident 15 years ago, which "was her fault" and resulted in the crushing of all her facial bones. She notes that facial pain is still significant as are migraines. She adds that she cannot tolerate any degree of pain due to her previous accident. She becomes tearful when describing her past history of incurring a fractured ankle on the left 6 years ago. When describing her life in the past, she is tearful, especially when explaining that she lost two children in childbirth.

Occupational therapy was recommended five times per week for 4 weeks to include achieving an optimal level of independence in ADL, independence in bed mobility and sitting balance for functional tasks, attendance and performance in a cooking group, and incorporation of her knitting into her therapeutic programming as well as relaxation techniques.

Obstacles encountered were her extreme response to pain, which inhibited any movement, extreme anticipation of pain, tearfulness, frequent complaints about the facility (regarding food, size of her room, and so forth) and, in general, her oppositional attitude toward therapeutic programming. She would frequently shriek with any slight bodily movement and would instruct therapists on the most optimal way in which to position her body or to transfer her, or would direct the pace and sequencing of the treatment session. She continued with complaints of facial and ankle pain (injuries many years prior) when sessions became difficult. Often, it appeared she used these complaints to stall or circumvent the task at hand. The patient was minimally responsive to refocusing, but the therapist noted that if she was given several minutes, the patient would be ready to continue to work. When she was not the focus of full attention, her somatic complaints or difficult behaviors escalated.

The therapist must decide how to acknowledge the patient's feelings of discomfort for her knee and validate her feelings of lost independence while instructing the patient on proper weight-shift techniques. The therapist must also decide how to provide a nurturing environment with an effective protocol while protecting other therapists from her hostile, accusatory behaviors.

—Marianne Fung, OTR/L

Answer

Mrs. X. is a survivor. Even though she was abandoned by one husband, lost two children in childbirth, and has experienced severe physical pain, she has remarried, raised six children, supported her family, achieved mastery in special interests, and developed a dependable social support network. She is the "comeback kid." Her character is resilient in the face of emotional and physical pain; but she still needs to acknowledge and express her pain and to receive nurturing. She can be exhorted to use the capacities that she used when faced with past challenges to persevere in the current challenge of rehabilitation and to speed exit from treatment (her stated goal).

The goal of motivational intervention is to help Mrs. X. determine how she can quickly exit rehabilitation.

The first intervention strategy would be to acknowledge Mrs. X.'s pain and the difficult challenges of rehabilitation that are made more challenging by her pain history. To the extent possible (i.e, without compromising rehabilitation), incorporate her suggestions for the least painful ways to position her and to pace and sequence therapy. Next, point out her tremendous successes in overcoming personal challenges throughout her life and ask her how she managed those situations. Try to identify useful qualities and traits that she can access for this new challenge. Help Mrs. X. take charge of developing strategies to reach her goal of quick exit from rehabilitation (e.g., repeatedly probing "What can you and I do to speed your exit from rehabilitation?") to help her arrive at concrete plans that can be jointly implemented.

Help Mrs. X. develop functional goals (involving use of her knee) related to her most valued interests (e.g., cooking, socializing, knitting). These interests give a meaningful context to the grueling rehabilitation tasks she has to perform. Ask her to visualize doing the most important of these tasks and to think of a word or phrase that will call this image to mind. This cue can help her envision successful performance of the task and refocus her during the painful moments in therapy. This may also help Mrs. X. envision the needed functional skills involved in her valued activities.

Encourage use of relaxation techniques before therapy in the evenings. This can help her not only relax but also get restorative sleep, which will bolster her for the next day's rehabilitation efforts. Check to see if she is getting restful sleep; pain may be interfering with truly restorative sleep. Mild medications may be needed for this. Finally, encourage her to reward herself and relax with a valued, richly meaningful activity after the day's rehabilitation. Knitting could serve this purpose.

Mrs. X.'s behaviors in rehabilitation (e.g., instructing therapists on how to position her body; not responding to refocusing, but informing therapists that she would regain her focus momentarily) suggest that she needs to have more control of the process. Her extreme response to pain and its anticipation simply need to be acknowledged (if the pain is not acknowledged, she will make it known) as legitimate and worthy of consideration. Mrs. X. is getting the reputation (her identity in this new environment) of attracting attention in negative ways like shrieking in pain. She could counterbalance this image, relax, and add greater, more realistic, and satisfying dimension to her identity in this setting by participating in her highly successful hobby and work interest of knitting.

With help developing plans and ways to cope with the pain of rehabilitation, emphasis on the need to prepare for the extreme effort and pain of treatment, and help attending to her overall wellness, Mrs. X. will gain more control of the process. By getting restorative sleep, relaxing, and balancing the extreme efforts with the personally validating and symbolically rewarding performance of valued and mastered activities (e.g., knitting, which may also garner her some social recognition), Mrs. X. may help to manage her pain, learn new stress management skills, and gain comfort and recognition from her strengths. This approach will sustain her through the difficult process of rehabilitation.

—*Janet H. Watts, MS, OTR/C*

◆　　◆　　◆

BALKING AT DISCHARGE: DEPRESSED, DEPENDENT, DISENGAGED

This 68-year-old woman, a widow of 12 years, was admitted to the acute care inpatient mental health unit of a general hospital with a diagnosis of major depression. This patient was 1 year post-right CVA and an ex-smoker, with a diagnosis of chronic obstructive pulmonary disease (COPD) times 4 years. Recent symptoms included decreased sleeping, eating, and motivation and lowered physical tolerance. The patient lived alone in her own home and received supports from VNA and home health aides (times 8 months).

Prior to retirement at age 64, the patient had a long career as an executive secretary. She married at age 35 and had no children. She had many friends from former working years and prior to the CVA had enjoyed eating out and playing cards with friends. The patient took pride in her career accomplishments and her former company. Family supports include a niece who lives 50 miles from the patient.

The patient was a well-groomed woman who moved slowly and sometimes appeared slow in understanding. She scored 5.2 on the Allen Cognitive Level Test. At the time of admission, she was alert, oriented, articulate, and was able to dress herself and do personal hygiene activities. She received moderate assistance in bathing, showering, and shampooing. The patient stated that she quickly fatigued while performing these activities. The patient also received help with home management, including budgeting, bill paying, and shopping. The patient drove her own car until 1 week prior to admission. She watched television during her leisure time, listened to music, and played Scrabble with volunteers.

The patient appeared to have little belief in her own ability to regain strength or to become more independent in self-care. She expressed no interest in resuming prior social activities and was anxious about her ability to continue to live alone. The only goal she expressed for herself was to build up stamina to walk to the end of the driveway to collect her own mail. The patient appeared dependent and in need of support and reassurance.

The occupational therapy goals and plans for the patient are that the patient will demonstrate increased stamina and muscle strength and she will note the improvement. To accomplish this goal, the patient will attend daily the Stretch and Relax Group, the baking group, and the therapeutic crafts group, where she will work on projects to increase upper extremity ROM and muscle strength. The patient will identify three areas of priority for improvement in ADL. She will list three strategies for increased participation in home management and will set short-term and long-term goals for home management. The patient will attend Life Skills Group. She will identify her own interests, skills, strengths, and values and will plan two ways to increase social contacts after discharge. She will also attend Expressive Therapy Groups, Self-Esteem Group, and Leisure Planning Group.

The patient attended occupational therapy groups consistently during admission. She was often dependent on other patients and enlisted them in her aid. She showed minimal improvement in belief in own ability. She appeared to enjoy social contacts and support of fellow patients.

At time of the patient's evaluation for discharge and return to independent living, it became evident her abilities, including mental status, cognitive level, coordination, and judgment did not concur with her level of confidence or her self-assessment of her ability to manage in her own home. The patient did not feel ready for discharge nor able to successfully function at home. The therapist's problem was to clarify the patient's discharge goals and to determine the most appropriate disposition.

—*Virginia Smith, OTR/L*

Answer

If one is to address the occupational therapists' concerns related to clarifying the discharge goals of this patient and determining the most appropriate discharge plan, considerably more information is necessary. Discerning relevant motivational and intervention processes and goals will require obtaining information that expands and adds depth and dimension to what is currently available in this clinical vignette.

Certainly, motivation is a principal issue and until that dynamic is tapped, prognosis will be limited. Self-initiated identification of interests and abilities is most often impossible during a depression and this expectation many times adds to the patient's sense of hopelessness. Similarly, the goal of resuming prior social activities is too frightening and challenging for her at this time. Such engagement requires more energy than she can generate now and would point up the difference between her abilities then and now. This woman's expressed fear about living alone, furthermore, shows how vulnerable and inadequate she feels. Thus, it is critical at this juncture for her to succeed in an activity commensurate with her current capabilities and previous values. Perhaps, for example, her demonstrated interest in Scrabble could be used to provide a sense of mastery and as a bridge to other word games and puzzles that would verify her ability. Such activity could then provide the context for nonthreatening social engagement. Are there other skills and previous interests that can be tapped and accommodated to her current capacities to elicit the motivation that will be necessary for her to move beyond her here and now? What information is needed for such discovery?

The fundamental question is what will engage this woman? For the depressed person especially, it is the past that holds the motivational trigger. Today and tomorrow are bleak. It is therefore important to understand what activities, done with whom, have characterized her way of living prior to her illness, how she describes these, and what has had meaning for her.

Motivation is triggered and sustained when there is congruence, a match, between the characteristics of an activity and the biopsychosocial characteristics and culture of the person. Discovering what will elicit motivation is a shared journey between the occupational therapist and the patient. It calls into play the art and the science of occupational therapy and evolves through dialogue between the two, supplemented by assessment findings as well as collaboration, in this instance, with the social worker and others who can help round out a profile of this woman.

Some of the questions that would guide such a profile would include

- What activities characterized her lifestyle prior to her marriage? Were these continued after her marriage?

- What activities did she and her husband share? How would she describe these? Were they (she) involved in community activities such as church, clubs, organizations? What did these activities include? Were these activities continued after the death of her husband? How did his death change her activities and way of living? What activities did she pursue on her own? How were these meaningful for her?

- What about special friendships? What activities did she share with friends? How frequently? What was most enjoyable about these? Least enjoyable?

- What about her hobbies? What is or was her favorite music? Preferred television program? What kind of card games did she enjoy? What does she remember most about her career? What was most enjoyable? Least enjoyable? How does she describe the company for which she worked? How difficult was it for her to leave? To adjust to retirement? What work relationships were continued after retirement? In what ways?

- How does she describe the ways in which her stroke and respiratory difficulties have changed her way of living? Before her depression, what activities could she do? Want to do? Has she found managing her home and living alone difficult? In what ways?

This woman has experienced several serious losses in the last 12 years—her husband, her career, and the decline of her health. The psychological and physical changes associated with these traumas make the depth of her depression and her fear of independence understandable. Knowing more about her will help provide the clues for tapping her unique strengths, capacities, and past interests to ensure successful endeavors and guard against threatening challenges, at least until a returning sense of competence and intrinsic motivation begins to emerge. It seems reasonable to expect that knowing more about her previous activity patterns would lead to finding ways congruent with her current physical and psychological state, for example, using her skills of engaging others and of eliciting their help, or demonstrating her past work competence through contributions to a substitute or surrogate "company."

Certainly the reality of her physical health must be a consideration in setting both short-term and discharge goals. Having a reasonably clear perspective of the impact of her depression versus the realistic limitations resulting from the CVA and COPD will indeed influence establishing relevant goals and lifestyle adjustments.

How limiting is her respiratory disease? What treatment is she receiving? What limitations exist as a result of the CVA? Is she currently receiving occupational or physical therapy?

Additionally, the question of her living arrangements must be addressed. Is living alone a prudent long-term goal for this woman? If engagement with others is important for her, are there easily available, regular social connections for her at home? Are there other arrangements that are more congruent with her long-term needs, interests, and capabilities?

Addressing these questions and concerns should go a long way toward designing an occupational therapy Life Style Profile and intervention plan for this woman and helping her evolve new personally satisfying patterns of living.

—Gail S. Fidler, OTR, FAOTA

◆　　◆　　◆

SAFETY SUFFERS: MOTIVATIONAL OR COGNITIVE LOSS?

B.S. is an 83-year-old widower who recently underwent surgery for a right below-knee amputation secondary to peripheral vascular disease. Past medical history includes osteoarthritis and insulin-dependent diabetes mellitus. He has lived alone in a ground-floor apartment in a housing complex for the elderly for the past 10 years and receives weekday lunches from Meals on Wheels. The patient has been discharged from a subacute facility and has returned to his home environment. Occupational therapy referral was received and ADL and home safety evaluations were requested. Current roles include father, grandfather, neighbor, retiree, and patient. B.S. is a retired steelworker who had been a foreman for 31 years. Previous interests included fishing, political campaigning, and participating in activities at the local Elks Lodge. B.S. was the primary caregiver for his wife, who had Parkinson's disease and died 3 years ago. The patient is unable to identify any current interests except for weekly visits from his young grandchildren. Three daughters live nearby and visit often and the patient also has a case manager who visits weekly.

B.S.'s goal is to be independent in ADL. He believes that he is doing well and does not really "need" therapy "because everything is just fine." Initial occupational therapy evaluation revealed that the patient was dependent in donning and doffing of prosthesis and bathing activities secondary to safety reasons. B.S. did not demonstrate safety awareness or good judgment during activities.

Occupational therapy goals for this patient are that he will be independent in bathing ADL with tub seat at seated level and in transferring on and off tub seat with his walker. Also, the patient will be independent in completing cold beverage and meal preparation at standing level with his walker.

Occupational therapy will visit B.S. two to three times a week for 5 weeks. Treatment approaches will include transfer training, meal preparation activities, functional tasks, patient education, prosthetic training, energy conservation techniques, and work simplification.

B.S. has not been compliant with medications and meals, so he is often disoriented due to uncontrolled blood sugar and is unable to participate in therapy. He insists on independent living but does not perform basic ADL to regulate medical needs. He is unaware of his behavior and its impact on his safety.

—*Joanne M. Gallagher, MS, OTR*

Answer

In order to understand the problems facing B.S., a number of questions and some supplemental information should be pursued. The first concern, perhaps, is to reach a better understanding of the extent to which his noncompliance relates to his need to deny the amputation of his leg and his declining health and to a developing cognitive deterioration. Certainly an amputation is traumatic and to come to some understanding of what this means to B.S. requires information about his previous lifestyle, self-concept, and values.

If denial plays a major role in his behavior, then motivation becomes the overriding focus in achieving compliance. If, on the other hand, a developing loss of cognitive functioning is a primary variable, then an appropriate program of cognitive mapping should be an initial concern. In all probability, B.S. struggles with a combination of each. An assessment of motor planning (AMP) would be helpful in gaining perspective relative to his current functioning. Additional personal data would give dimension to understanding this man's traditional lifestyle and what has characterized the gratifying experiences in his living.

This information should offer clues to arrive at those activities likely to trigger motivation that would lead to coping and compliance with the goals of more self-dependent functioning. For instance, if fishing were a serious interest, perhaps sharing in some aspect of the activity with a grandchild would trigger incentive. Or his previous campaigning activity, if this has truly been a previous skill and interest, could be adapted and related to current similar activities. Being a foreman in a steel mill for 31 years suggests some significant skills and values that should certainly provide clues to how this man can become reengaged in activity that will contribute to the quality of his life.

Some areas to pursue should include his experiences as a foreman and steel worker. How does he describe his job? His role as a foreman? What tasks were most enjoyable and rewarding? Which ones did he dislike? How does he describe his skills, his shortcomings?

How does he describe his role as a caretaker? What was most rewarding? What tasks did he dislike? What activities did he and his wife share? What have been his previous interests and hobbies? What type of fishing did he do? How frequently? What does he remember most about this? When did he stop fishing? Why? What was his campaigning activity about? How does he describe these experiences? Why has he not continued this activity? How was he involved with the Elks Lodge? What friends and activities were related to this affiliation?

What about friends? Did he or does he have many? A few? How does he describe his friendships? His acquaintances? Activities shared with friends in the past?

How old are his grandchildren? What can he tell us about them? Their interests? How does he or might he spend time with them? How does he describe his engagement with his daughters? What activities do they and have they shared?

The occupational therapy goals and their expectations can be achieved only if they are germane to B.S.'s cognitive and emotional capacities to cope and adapt. In our overriding concern for the quality of this man's life, we must ask what are his realistic strengths and capacities and what activity experience will trigger the motivational force necessary for moving toward a way of living, more satisfying than not, to himself and to others?

—*Gail S. Fidler, OTR, FAOTA*

◆   ◆   ◆

GRIEF AND THE BOTTLE

The patient is a 78-year-old, widowed male admitted for the fifth time to the secure psychiatric unit with a diagnosis of chronic alcohol use (times 60 years). His associated medical diagnosis is hearing loss secondary to loud machinery that requires use of a hearing aid. The patient was admitted to the inpatient unit by his daughter who lives outside New England. He has no other children and his wife of 50 years died 6 months ago.

Prior to admission, the patient had been living in a three-bedroom home for 20 years, unassisted, with no outside services provided. The patient receives Social Security and retirement benefits from 30 years of work as a conductor with the railroads. He reports that his only reason to leave home in the past 6 months has been to take a cab for errands and to walk to a few neighbors for visits. The patient elected to stop driving 4 years ago. He reports that he had previously been heavily dependent on his late wife's "running of the household." The patient assisted with laundry, trash, and basic cooking. The patient reports socializing daily while walking to the store in the town center and is well known around town. Before his wife's death, the patient enjoyed gardening and carpentry tasks.

The patient acknowledges he has always used whiskey to "lift my mood or to get away from it all." He is aware of the medical and psychiatric consequences, yet expresses minimal intention to curb his use. His remarks regarding use are, "I always have, why change now?" He does admit to severe depression since his wife's death.

On the fourth day following detoxification, the patient scored 4.6 on the Allen Cognitive Level Test. This score corresponds to observations of his personal hygiene and care and to the recent decline of handling basic home management tasks reported by his daughter.

The occupational therapy treatment plan is to address the patient's current and anticipated cognitive levels. To improve his cognitive status, the patient will complete one concrete task daily during therapeutic crafts group and he will note this improvement. The patient demonstrates a decline in the performance of self-care and ADL as evidenced by direct observation from family and staff. Therefore, the patient will review and list daily priorities with the occupational therapist to ensure appropriate attention is given to his needs, including personal safety. The patient will successfully perform these functions on the unit prior to discharge. The patient increasingly isolates himself and reports he has reduced his interactions with acquaintances. The short-term plan is to engage the patient in a one-on-one interaction and in a small group.

Major obstacles to this patient's treatment are his lack of desire to change and lack of belief in the ability to change his alcohol abuse. The patient neither works to improve ADL skills nor believes improved self-care to be possible.

The dilemma for the occupational therapist is how to engage the patient to make efforts to improve functioning? What discharge planning would be in the patient's best interest?

—*Marcy Lee, OTR/L*

Answer

The patient's nuclear problem is the death of his wife and unresolved grief issues surrounding her death. I do not see the alcohol as nuclear but contributory to his hospitalization, because he has been an alcoholic for over 60 years. This abuse has been chronic and the primary admission this time revolves around his wife's death. His decline of ADL, social skills, and performance of other life tasks are directly related to her death. It seems that he has lost his "reason for living" and all meaningful things in life appear to have revolved around his wife and her being present. The patient even admits to depression since his wife's death; however, the grief issues may have been overlooked by many because he may have been labeled an alcoholic so "there's not much we can do here." Death and dying issues are not easy for anyone to discuss in our culture and are often overlooked by occupational therapists. It is vital to explore these issues with any patient, especially a patient like this one with this history. The issues need to be explored in the context of development and reinstatement of life skills, not as other health professionals might explore the issues to "talk it through." Talking it through to more understanding of the problem is positive but is not the primary domain of an occupational therapist. We must always work toward more positive engagement in occupations with concrete observations made to that end.

In this case, the plan of care does not reflect the patient's unresolved grief, because, if his reason for living is gone, why get dressed in the morning? Why socialize with mutual friends of 50 years (sometimes it is more painful than positive)? So, interacting with strangers and performing ADL just to perform it for a therapist can be as meaningless as his life seems right now. To restore meaning, exploration of death and dying issues, grief, what his wife meant to him, and the life they shared and built together can all be positive and meaningful activities that will then facilitate engagement in life tasks. The patient needs to find tasks that provide meaning for him for which it is worth getting up in the morning. Having the patient create a collage of their 50 years together could be positive. If he chooses to avoid discussions or projects involving his wife, create conversations that get to the life tasks that are meaningful right now or were in the past. Do an occupational history to uncover former interests, coping styles (we know alcohol was one coping style), and life goals and dreams. Perhaps his goals and dream was to marry, have children, and lead a good

life. He has done that. So, a possibility is that no support group, therapy treatments, or social and life task involvement will be beneficial to him at 78 years of age. There may be a need to allow him all the choices, exploring the costs and benefits of continued drinking and his maladaptive behaviors, along with exploring the benefits (which might be hard to see right now) of therapy, somewhat decreasing his drinking, using short-term medications, and getting his daughter more actively involved if possible. For a drinker of 60 years, the best we can possibly hope for is that he drinks a little less and in a safe environment. Lifeline support can be started.

Finally, his drinking started when he was 18 (according to the history). Other health services in collaboration with occupational therapy might be able to uncover why he never stopped, which might give clues to helping him now. He also states that he has little belief in himself or in improved task performance. Therefore, he may always have been dependent and has accomplished little in life of which to be proud. Perhaps he could engage in carpentry and gardening skills for his wife's memorial, planting her favorite flower at her grave site. If he wants to avoid the death, perhaps he could make small objects and plant minigardens for sick children or for neighbors. The occupational therapist could involve his neighbors and community, as well as his daughter, and have them request things to be made, going so far as to keep him company (if that is acceptable with him) while he creates. Increasing activity level will help with grief work, along with medications and some psychotherapy, if he will cooperate. But the major intervention, I feel, is to uncover past reasons for his behavior so the therapist has an understanding. The therapist can then develop grief work activities and get other disciplines involved, involve others the patient knows and loves, and open conversation to be honest regarding the costs and benefits of his drinking and other maladaptive behaviors. If the patient chooses to continue with his present actions, discharge planning can be to a safe environment where his needs are taken care of. Otherwise a great potential exists for reclusive and unsafe behaviors if he should live alone. A community watch (since he was so well liked) could have neighbors visit, a different one each day, and go out for a meal or bring one in; get the church or synagogue involved; have neighbor children visit and ask him to plant flowers or make something for them. This will help him to be safer and feel important enough to someone to carry on.

—*Michael Pizzi, MS, OTR/L,*
CHES, FAOTA

◆　　◆　　◆

PAIN MANAGEMENT IS THE KEY

E.J. is an 86-year-old, widowed female who recently sustained a fracture of the neck of the left femur and underwent open reduction and internal fixation surgery to stabilize the fracture. Past medical history includes orthostatic hypotension, epilepsy, and hypothyroidism. E.J. has returned to her home after a 3-week stay in a subacute facility and intends to resume independent living in her second-floor apartment in a housing complex for the elderly. Prior to her fall, she was independent in all activities of daily living. Her life roles include mother, grandmother, homemaker, neighbor, and patient. She is a retired elementary schoolteacher and Bible study leader. Her social interests include weekly bridge and bingo games held in her housing complex. She is in contact with one of her two surviving children, her one son, who lives 3 hours away and visits each Saturday.

E.J.'s goal was to be independent in all ADL, primarily tub seat transfers and bathing. She believed that she would progress through her rehabilitative program if she worked hard and followed through with the therapists' recommendations. She realized her seizures could occur without warning and had made appropriate lifestyle changes, such as employing Lifeline support and allowing neighbors access to her apartment for routine observations.

The occupational therapy goals for E.J. are that she will be able to transfer independently on and off the tub seat with her walker and will be able to complete bathing independently with the tub seat for two sessions. E.J. will be able to independently dress her lower extremities using adaptive equipment at a seated level. She will also be able to independently complete cold and hot meal preparation at a standing level with a walker.

Occupational therapy visits are

scheduled for two to three times a week for 4 weeks. Treatment approaches include patient education, transfer training, adaptive equipment, compensatory techniques, meal preparation activities, and energy conservation techniques.

E.J. participates in treatment occasionally but often refuses secondary to pain. She is unable to work "through" the pain and prefers not to perform, but she realizes that compliance with therapy is necessary for improvement.

The patient is not progressing with occupational therapy goals. E.J. refuses elder care services, which would provide meal preparation and light homemaking duties, and she may be unsafe in her home environment. Her performance in therapy is poor and in conflict with her personal goals.

—*Joanne M. Gallagher, MS, OTR/L*

Answer

E.J.'s main problem is, on the surface, a hip fracture. The occupational therapy recommendations, plan of care, and goals are all very appropriate. What appears to be a nuclear problem affecting her is how to cope with pain. E.J. appears motivated and wishes to do the "right thing," but she is limited by her inability to cope with pain.

Before we proceed with the pain issue, I would also ask some questions regarding her fall. It seems she fell because of an epileptic seizure, and she has made lifestyle changes to adapt to that problem. However, she still lives on a second floor, which is unsafe for someone who experiences seizures.

Given her pain, she should be on a first floor in an assisted living arrangement. She can also move in with a son if, indeed, this is a feasible choice.

Pain is a factor in life that demands closer observation and analysis and cannot be simplified, resulting in therapists giving up or prematurely discharging patients. Clinically, we often are confronted with pain as an issue but do not have clinical, educational, or even practical resources at our fingertips to assist us in using sound clinical reasoning to help with pain management and facilitate independent living. Indeed, we often do not have any basic training in pain-management activities or techniques and often must rely on continuing education and other training. In E.J.'s case, if pain is not resolved, it could lead to permanent disability and affect future living arrangements that she might not desire. I feel the pain issue is a major reason for the lack of motivation, and it can be multifactorial.

Let us explore some of the factors for the pain and some exacerbating reasons for pain.

1. Physical pain is real, and weight bearing on her left leg is difficult for her to cope with.

2. Her son lives 3 hours away. Can pain be a way of gaining his attention and getting him to help her problem solve a way out of her dilemma? Certainly, we must know or at least be aware of the family dynamics so we can rule out that the pain is a family dynamic.

3. Note that the case study states she is in contact with only one son of two surviving children. This must say

something about loss of relationships and how the pain may be related to that loss.

4. Perhaps E.J. is what I call a chronic whiner. This is a person who, no matter what the positive experiences are in life, "whines" about how bad things are. Whining is simply a way to get attention and a form of communication that is maladaptive if it persists. Therapists need to explore the reasons for that form of communicating and determine if E.J. has been a whiner all her life.

5. Perhaps the pain is exacerbated by the possibility that she feels out of control and has few choices in her treatment program.

No matter the reasons, E.J. is experiencing pain, perceived or real. This is affecting her life performance and development of skills that will directly affect her living situation. She is experiencing conflict between her personal goals and achievements and her reasons for nonachievement. I believe that direct and honest communication between the therapist and E.J. could benefit her greatly by engaging her in pain management through conversation about the pain issue. I also suggest that the therapist explore some wellness techniques and alternatives to pain management besides positioning and energy conservation, such as techniques that include relaxation, deep breathing, and imagery while involved in functional tasks. E.J. has some hobbies she can do while standing that can be more fully explored. She could bake a cake for her visiting son, too. Use the family dynam-

ic issue positively as a motivator, and have E.J. make short-term progress to show her son the next weekend. Using an interdisciplinary team approach may also benefit E.J. Other staff may have pain-management techniques they can show the occupational therapist or use with E.J. if they are on the team.

—*Michael Pizzi, MS, OTR/L,*
CHES, FAOTA

◆　　◆　　◆

DYING IS "NO LONGER DOING"

During the course of our careers as occupational therapists, many of us may encounter the situation of treating a patient who is dying, whether it be from a terminal illness or "old age." It is helpful for us as therapists to understand the various stages these patients may experience. Dr. Elizabeth Kubler-Ross describes these stages as "denial and isolation, anger, bargaining, depression, and acceptance" (Hopkins & Smith, 1993, p. 855). The dying patient may fluctuate among any of these stages at any given time during the dying process, using either adaptive or maladaptive behaviors based on his or her interactions with the environment.

It is sometimes difficult to know exactly what our role as occupational therapist is with the dying patient. During the past 2 of my 13 years as a certified occupational therapy assistant, I have worked in a subacute nursing and rehabilitation center. Recently, I worked with a patient who had been diagnosed a few months prior with lung cancer with metastasis to the brain. This 66-year-old, married man had led an active and productive life as a firefighter in a major city and had two daughters and one son. When admitted to our facility, it was with the understanding that he was to be discharged home when his condition had stabilized. To accomplish this goal, our therapy sessions focused on improved strength and endurance, safety issues, and daily living skills. We also focused on leisure activities, such as watercolor painting, which had been important to him prior to his illness, and adapted them to his present physical capabilities. Unexpectedly, though, his condition began to deteriorate rapidly. He became depressed, not wanting to leave his room, eat, or take his medication. The nursing staff asked that I speak to him (as we had established a good rapport) and try to encourage him to eat and take his medication.

During the course of our conversation, I began to understand why he was refusing to take his medication. He described to me how "his body felt like it was going to die and his brain was telling him he was going to die but his heart was not ready." The medication made him confused and disoriented and his "time was too precious to spend in confusion."

We sat in his room and he began reminiscing about the various roles in which he had functioned during his lifetime, as a father, husband, firefighter, and friend. He told me how much difficulty he was having at relinquishing these roles and how much more he wanted to do. We talked about the meaning these roles held for him and the impact

he had on other people's lives. I was able to reassure him of the value of his life based on conversations I had with various family members and friends.

Toward the end of our conversation, my patient asked if I would hug him. I sat on the edge of the bed and held him while he cried, trying to maintain my own composure and remain "professional." We stayed like this until his wife arrived, and, after speaking briefly to her, I left the room.

My patient died the next day at the age of 66. I grieved for him even though I had only known him for a month, and I grieved for the loss his family was feeling. While I understood my role as a therapist during our treatment sessions that focused on the physical aspects of his illness, I questioned my role as his therapist during this last stage of his life.

Marcil and Tigges wrote a book entitled *Terminal and Life Threatening Illness: An Occupational Behavior Perspective* (1988), which helped to clarify my roles for me. The authors stressed the importance of an individual's self-concept, which makes that person unique, and the impact that a physical illness or disease has on the components of self-concept. Health professionals frequently focus on the physical problems of the patient rather than on the total person. Attention to and care of the symptoms of the disease will not save the dying person's life. Therapists need to pay attention to the patient's physical condition, yet careful attention also needs to be given to the patient's personhood, allowing the therapist to "bring a sense of safety, security, and well being in the final months, weeks, or days of life" (Marcil & Tigges, 1988, p. 92).

Mark Rosenfeld is a professor at Worcester State College where I am finishing my Bachelor's degree. He also helped me to define my role as a therapist in his situation. Apparently, I had helped my patient understand the meaning and beauty of his life and helped him to see the powerful effect he had on other lives. I believe that I helped my patient to die with dignity in a way that was appropriate for him, without medication or heroic efforts. He was able to maintain a sense of control over his life and death. I feel honored that he wanted me to share in this final stage of his life.

As occupational therapists, we can help our patients who are dying give meaning to their life and death. To do this well, we must recognize that reflecting on the meaning of past functioning can be valuable even when further doing is impossible. Occupational therapy addresses the performance and patterns of work, leisure, chores, and rest. Just as relaxation and sleep must be included in the context of every day, so is death a rest that can be integrated at the end of every life. While I, like many occupational therapists, am a productivity-oriented person, I now believe that we should strive to understand and incorporate "not doing" into our practice. To do this, we must embrace rest, sleep, and even death as elements of our domain of concern and further develop occupational strategies related to these areas of life.

—*Cindy Kennealy, COTA/L, OTS*

References

Hopkins, H.L., & Smith, H.D. (1993). *Willard and Spackman's occupational therapy* (8th ed.). Philadelphia: Lippincott.

Marcil, W.M., & Tigges, K.N. (1988). *Terminal and life threatening illness: An occupational behavior perspective.* Thorofare, NJ: Slack.

❖　　❖　　❖

A WIDOWER'S DILEMMA

Mr. S. is an 82-year-old, recently widowed male diagnosed with pneumonia, depression, and bladder cancer needing a Foley catheter, which he has had for approximately 2 years. He had been living in a housing complex for the elderly in Massachusetts for the past 15 years with his wife of 60 years until she passed away suddenly 3 months ago. Mr. S. is a retired fire captain. He took part in many activities, including the noon meal and the nightly discussion group in the Senior Center attached to the housing complex, and was a eucharistic minister at his church until he was diagnosed with cancer. His wife did most of the household chores and driving secondary to his decreased endurance. In the past, Mr. S. relied on his wife for emotional support and structure in his life and her death has been a very difficult adjustment. Mr. S. has one daughter who lives in Washington, D.C., who has been involved in setting up community services. Her relationship with her father has been strained for many years.

He was referred for home services following discharge from a skilled nursing facility after recovering from pneumonia. An occupational therapy referral was made after he was home for 3 weeks. At that time, he was receiving nursing services, mental health counseling, and physical therapy two times per week, and visits by a home-health aide two times per day. At this time he is being started on antidepressant medication.

During the occupational therapy evaluation, Mr. S. was unable to control his crying regarding the loss of his wife. He reminisced about the days in the hospital with her and his subsequent hospitalization in the room next door. He showed the therapist his 60th wedding anniversary pictures and a greeting they received from the Pope for this momentous occasion. At this time, Mr. S. stated his main goal was to stay in his own apartment and not go into a long-term-care facility; however, "if his daughter tells him to, he will."

Functionally, Mr. S. is independent in hygiene and grooming activities, dressing, toileting, and eating, though he does not initiate this without the home-health aide being present. He requires minimal assistance with tub transfers, bathing, handling his catheter, and light meal preparation. He uses a walker for mobility. He is within functional limits in ROM and strength, though endurance is fair. Cognitively, his safety, judgment, and short-term memory are minimally to moderately impaired; however, it is unclear if this is due to the depression or true cognitive decline.

Occupational therapy will meet with Mr. S. for 1 hour two to three times per week. The therapist will work with the home-health aide to encourage Mr. S. to do his self-care independently. Other occupational therapy goals are to increase Mr. S.'s independence in light meal preparation and in tub transfers, and to increase socialization skills.

After 2 weeks of treatment, Mr. S. continues to rely on the home-health aide to do his self-care and cries for half of the occupational therapy treatment session. He discusses relying on his daughter to take care of him, though she shows no interest in moving closer to him or having him move closer to her. How does the therapist help this patient work through this crisis and help him to achieve his goal of staying in his own apartment with support?

—*Cheryl Lucas, MS, OTR/L*

Answer

Mr. S. is clearly in crisis over the death of his wife, his primary support both emotionally and functionally. This depression has led to his inability to care adequately for himself. He also is unable to problem solve ways to take control of his life and function independently with help from community supports. His sadness regarding being placed in a nursing home and yet his compliance, i.e., "whatever my daughter says, I will do," has left Mr. S. hopeless and helpless, with an inability to see his strengths and plan for the future.

The goals of motivational intervention are to help Mr. S. acknowledge the loss of his wife, become accustomed to his new role as a widower, and become aware of his strengths in the functional skills that will allow him to remain in his familiar environment.

Several specific intervention strategies were identified to help Mr. S. meet his goal. The occupational therapist will help Mr. S. set up a daily routine. This would include blocks of time to do tasks he needs to accomplish in order to live independently at home. The schedule should coincide with times and activities he is familiar with. For example, dressing should not come first, if he usually eats and has coffee before he dresses. Included in this daily routine should be self-care, light homemaking (making a bed), light meal preparation, and socialization activities. The next strategy is to break down the tasks of the schedule and assess the activities Mr. S. can and cannot do. Schedule therapy time during daily routines to practice activities he cannot do independently, for example, shower and tub transfer at 8:00 a.m., catheter care at 9:00 a.m., if that is when the home-health aide is scheduled. Help Mr. S. schedule lunch at the Senior Center instead of having the home-health aide prepare it. Work on building endurance to get there, meal preparation for one meal, as well as accessing community resources.

Encourage Mr. S. to reconnect socially with people he was friendly with in the church and Senior Center. The nightly discussion group he and his wife participated in would be a good start, as he knows the people who participate and would be welcomed. During a treatment session, walk to the Senior Center to find out times of activities he likes, for example, church services or discussion groups. Work on compiling a list of community resources. Have Mr. S. use a telephone book or other directory to list transportation services, physician numbers, homemaker services, and church-friendly visitors.

These tasks were chosen to help Mr. S. regain a sense of himself as a hopeful, self-reliant individual with resources to get help if needed. By taking part in occupational therapy treatment, Mr. S. gets the opportunity to use skills he has and to learn new skills when necessary. The activities chosen help to sustain occupational patterns and involvement by returning to a daily routine of activities he has done for many years and that have meaning to him. Occupational therapy treatment also involved teaching Mr. S. new skills like preparing light meals and organizing resources to help himself (cleaning services, doctor appointments, transportation), and adjusting to his role as a widower. By becoming active in the Senior Center, Mr. S. has an opportunity to reminisce about the activities he and his wife would do together. By taking part in the nightly informal discussion group, he can participate with others who knew his wife and also get involved in other discussions, especially with residents who might be widowers.

By participating in a daily routine, mastering his self-care skills, and participating daily in social activities, Mr. S. will be able to decrease his dependence on the home-care agency and increase his self-reliance to achieve his goal of staying in the apartment he has known for 15 years, thereby symbolizing recovery.

—Cheryl Lucas, MS, OTR/L

◆　　◆　　◆

CULTURAL TRADITIONS: OBSTACLE OR OPPORTUNITY?

Mr. A. is a 69-year-old, Asian male with a diagnosis of CVA, right hemiplegia, aphasia, and three previous CVAs with left hemiparesis. Mr. A. is married, with four very supportive children. He and his wife are living with the eldest son and daughter-in-law (according to Chinese customs) in a small, two-bedroom apartment. Prior to his return home in Texas, Mr. A. was in a hospital in Maryland receiving intensive inpatient rehabilitation. Upon the patient's return home, his physician ordered home care for nursing, physical, occupational, and speech therapies.

Mr. A. is a retired computer engineer, who prior to the CVA would travel and visit his children and grandchildren. He used to enjoy watching Chinese movies and reading the Chinese newspaper.

Mr. A. is currently dependent for all ADL and exhibits poor balance with severe spasticity in all four extremities, trunk, and facial musculature. He is expressively aphasic and appears to inconsistently comprehend simple one- or two-step commands.

As Mr. A. is unable to communicate to set goals, the family's goals were to keep him home, functioning at the highest level possible, and to independently and safely handle the patient for completion of ADL.

Mr. A.'s family appeared to be overwhelmed initially when he returned home. They lacked knowledge in proper positioning, ADL, transfers, proper and safe equipment, safety issues, home exercise program, and overall handling of the patient.

The family appeared fairly realistic regarding goals and the patient's abilities. Mrs. A. appeared to accept that the patient required assistance for all ADL and that it was her "duty" to "serve" him. Mrs. A. would spend her entire day "doing" for her husband.

Mr. A. was initially seen three times a week in conjunction with a physical therapist to safely handle the patient. Occupational therapy goals were established to train the caregivers in safe and independent handling of the patient, to obtain appropriate equipment and adaptive aids to maximize patient's independence and safety, and to establish a home exercise program for the patient's family to safely carry over with the patient to maximize his function.

Mr. A.'s level of motivation was initially poor, secondary to his lack of understanding and what was thought to be a cultural barrier. The family thought that since both therapists were female, the patient might be having a difficult time coping with the fact that two women were in a position of "authority." Mr. A. also appeared to get along better with the physical therapist, who is Caucasian, versus the occupational therapist, who is Chinese. Mr. A. would try and bite the therapists when he was stretched or when ROM was performed. Mr. A. eventually learned that after his exercises, he was more relaxed and could do more with his left arm.

The therapist's problem was the difficulty in always knowing what Mr. A.

was thinking and how to relate to him. The family was very supportive and had good carryover of the exercises they could actually do with the patient. It was hard for them to effectively stretch and range Mr. A. without the patient getting upset or angry.

—Janice Walker, OTR

Answer

The patient described in this clinical vignette presents a constellation of concerns that require the therapist to step back to contemplate the soundness of common treatment objectives. As occupational therapists, we orient our goals toward independent living and quality-of-life issues. At times, we confront a situation that challenges our creativity and impedes our progress toward those goals.

Mr. A. lives with his eldest son, as is Chinese custom. Concomitant cultural expectations would include a preference toward male caretakers, with the primary responsibility for guardianship resting with the eldest son (Chin Prince, 1996). The wife's role would be to generally "serve" her husband but not necessarily to make demands upon him, such as requiring his tolerance of painful stretching exercises.

Mr. A. has been an independent man, with a successful vocation and a penchant for traveling to connect with his offspring and maintain his patriarchal role. He is now confronted with considerable deficits that restrict his ability to sustain these previous occupations and symbolically challenge his position as head of the family. His attempts at regaining control are seen as resistance to intervention, and he is labeled a difficult patient.

Considering the cultural mores ingrained in this situation, occupational therapy would be oriented toward family support (as has already been stated) to sustain the members' connection with a minimum amount of additional stress via external demands and to provide some opportunity for Mr. A. to exercise limited control. The acceptance of family member roles (i.e., wife as server, son as intervener) would demonstrate acquiescence to the patient's needs despite our own view that the wife may have more time or availability to perform exercises or treatments. Equipment (air splints, series casts) that would maintain or increase range in a time frame acceptable to the patient rather than uncomfortable stretching sessions with a family member would partly remove the challenge to Mr. A.'s dignity. Of equal importance, the admission by home care therapists that comfort within cultural boundaries is acceptable would provide the family and the respective therapists with a more reasonable sense of accomplishment. For the patient, some return of previous leisure pursuits would allow a revisitation to better times. The inclusion of Chinese films, taped radio programming, or a relative reading the newspaper with him would provide a calming atmosphere during which time a splint could be applied or worn, or an exercise routine performed. Similar surroundings during nontreatment times would also allow Mr. A. to hold onto his central position in the family as leader, rather than merely being receiver of service due to his physical limitations.

—*Jacqueline R. Brennan, RPT/L,*
MS, OTR/L

Reference

Chin Prince, D. (April 8, 1996). Personal conversation.

◆   ◆   ◆

WITHDRAWING INWARD

This 94-year-old, never-married female was admitted to a rehabilitation and long-term-care facility as a long-term-care resident. The primary precipitant for admission was the woman's being unable to live independently due to the inability to perform ADL, including cooking, toileting, and bathing.

This woman has a medical history of osteoarthritis of the right knee and hypertension. The osteoarthritis has caused her to be wheelchair bound, thereby impeding her mobility. Other complications include diverticulosis, breast cancer, glaucoma, and a history of right wrist and right hip fracture.

This independent woman had lived alone in her two-bedroom apartment. Her primary life roles were taking care of her elderly mother and working as a nurse in various settings. This woman was very friendly and socially active in her community. Social activities included going out to lunch, shopping, and traveling with friends. She was also very active in her local church. She visited and brought food to the sick, made clothes for the poor, and taught the Bible to other members of her congregation. Her nursing career not only

supported her financially but also served as a social context that enabled her to meet and become friends with many people. She stated that her one regret in life was never having married, because now she does not have her own children to take care of her.

Currently she has a 72-year-old niece who visits her three times per week and a limited number of friends who visit her occasionally, especially around the holidays.

The patient is realistic regarding her illness; she understands and accepts decreased abilities due to the aging process. Unfortunately, the limitations the aging process has imposed on the patient may have resulted in her drawing inward and disengaging from society. This once very social and independent woman has limited her goals to the most basic life dignity: going to the toilet independently. The patient expresses that she feels "stupid" by not being able to accomplish such an apparently easy task. She appears to believe that rehabilitation will eventually lead to her goal but, unfortunately, she becomes easily discouraged by the amount of effort it takes. Does this discouraged attitude reflect her true feelings regarding her disability or are there deeper, underlying reasons for her demeanor, including her self-criticism?

The patient becomes easily discouraged when faced with adversity. She copes by accepting the disability as part of the natural aging process.

The patient's primary goal for occupational therapy is to toilet independently. The patient receives occupational therapy services three times per week for 45-minute sessions. The patient uses a wheelchair for mobility to the bathroom and safety bars to aid in transferring from the wheelchair to the toilet. The therapist works on upper extremity strength and endurance to allow the patient to transfer from the chair to the toilet.

The patient initially presents with a high motivational level, but during the treatment process she becomes easily discouraged and requests frequent assistance. Is this rapid discouragement due to actual life contentment and acceptance of the illness or is this a sign that the patient is disengaging from life?

The therapist's problem is to increase the actual motivational level of the patient as opposed to the perceived motivational level the patient verbalizes and to discover the underlying reasons for the patient's motivational difficulties.

—*Patty Pierce, OTS*

Answer

The patient has had a long, successful life characterized by independence, nurturance for others, and many varied social activities. Currently, she is dependent, has no opportunities to care for others, and has limited social contacts. The patient expresses self-criticism and regrets not having had children to care for her. Her stated goal is independent toileting, yet she is easily discouraged when working toward this goal.

The therapist observes the patient's easy discouragement and self-criticism and interprets these as indicating possible disengagement and passive acceptance of disability. The therapist also

has nagging concerns that she may not fully understand the patient's true feelings. I agree, suspect mild depression, and wonder if the patient's current situation (with functional limitations and disability) blocks need fulfillment (e.g., for independence, to help others, and to be involved with others). The observed acceptance and disengagement could be by default, as easy ways to adjust to losses (even though they may not allow for need fulfillment). The patient may accept limited visits, dependence, and lack of opportunities to give to others because she feels powerless to change things; thus, she may see acceptance and disengagement as her only dignified options. It is easier to accept a loss than take on the challenge of finding new ways to express her identity; however, this solution leaves the patient with the prospect of living the remainder of her life emotionally stifled. She may not believe that her current environment will acknowledge or support her efforts to stay meaningfully engaged.

I also wonder if the patient has an unmet need for nurturance? Does she need help (and permission) to explore what she needs as separate from what she may think others want for her? Is her self-chosen goal of independent toileting a socially desirable one that has shallow meaning or potency for her? (The easy discouragement may signal this.) The nuclear problem may be the patient's limited opportunities to explore and meet her needs and express her identity.

The goal of motivational intervention is to help discover the patient's true needs and wishes.

One intervention strategy is to provide nurturing. Show interest in understanding the patient's needs and wishes and show unconditional positive regard for her views. Observe her response to increased nurturing and support to determine if this is meeting a need. If she accepts the concern, if it helps her discuss her needs and wishes, and if it seems to help her comfortably be herself, it is meeting a need. Help her when she is discouraged, note the contrast between her goal and easy discouragement, suggest that this may signal a lack of interest in the task, and ask if this is something she truly wants to do now in therapy. The second intervention strategy is to facilitate discussion. Talk to the patient about her losses and brainstorm ways to regain a degree of need fulfillment. Possibly, provide a perspective that others in the facility are likely to have similar feelings. Explore ways to create and participate in social opportunities in the facility. The third intervention strategy is to encourage the patient. Offer suggestions for the patient to extend herself socially at the long-term-care facility (e.g., participate in crafts and discussion groups) for the purpose of exploring ways to help others (e.g., providing caring friendship or engaging in Bible study).

Nurturing for a short time may meet the patient's need to be cared for and help her comfortably explore other true needs (as opposed to socially desirable ones that may be unrelated to anything meaningful for the patient) and wishes. Nurturing may help the patient reengage socially, which can give purpose, meaning, and context to work on ADL, if she wants to. For example, she may be motivated to work on toileting independence if successful performance of this makes her more comfortable around other people. The social involvement may provide opportunities for her to help others as she did for a lifetime, providing a way to create continuity with the activities that constituted a meaningful life before long-term care. While she cannot provide physical assistance to others, nothing in her profile suggests any decline in mental abilities. Thus, she can draw on her experiences teaching the Bible and offering caring friendship to others.

This program of exploring true needs as a source of motivation may lead to activities that express the patient's identity, sustain meaningful involvement, and provide motivation and context for regaining functional skills.

—Janet H. Watts, MS, OTR/C

◆　　◆　　◆

HIGH ANXIETY IN A MEDICAL MINE FIELD

Mrs. N. is an 82-year-old, married female with a diagnosis of right CVA, macular degeneration, depression, hypothyroidism, and chronic anxiety disorder who is currently residing in a nursing and rehabilitation center. Mrs. N. was admitted to an acute care hospital for acute hemorrhagic right thalamus CVA and was transferred to this setting 2 weeks later for continuing rehabilitation. Prior to admission, Mrs. N. lived with her husband in a two-story home with the bedroom and bathroom on the second floor. The kitchen is on the first floor. Mrs. N. was independent with ADL and was the primary homemaker. Her major roles were wife, sister, and caregiver for her medically compromised husband. The family assisted with shopping, heavy housekeeping, and yard work. At the time of admission, Mrs. N. was unable to identify any leisure interests. With increased socialization, it was apparent that Mrs. N. enjoyed cooking and sharing past life experiences. On admission, Mrs. N. could self-feed, groom, upper extremity and lower extremity dress and bathe, and toilet with minimum assistance. Mrs. N. required moderate assistance to don bra and manage Depends. Mrs. N. could supine to sit, sit to stand, and transfer to functional surfaces with minimum assistance. Mrs. N. required minimum assistance to maintain sitting balance and required moderate assistance to maintain standing balance due to perceptual and proprioceptive problems. Maximum verbal and tactile cues were needed to motor plan all functional tasks. During the admission, the family visited and was generally supportive and involved in the discharge plans with some resistance from the husband.

Mrs. N. demonstrated her style of coping by the consistent statements that she wanted to return home but also made repeated statements of "I want to go to bed, I can't do this, and I'm so nervous." Mrs. N. slept poorly at night and also ate poorly. She exhibited constant hand wringing and frequent purposeless movement of hands and arms that interfered with functional activity. The family and Mrs. N. reported multi-

ple adversities in her history: left school to help raise family, previous psychiatric hospitalizations, and husband's failing health. Fifteen years ago, Mrs. N. was treated with electroconvulsive therapy with no improvement. At the present time, the family and Mrs. N. are resistant to inpatient psychiatric treatment recommended by the consulting psychiatrist.

Occupational therapy goals for Mrs. N. are that she will be able to

- feed herself independently 75% of a meal
- perform grooming independently from wheelchair level
- dress and bathe independently her upper and lower extremities after set-up
- transfer to bed and commode with supervision
- ambulate functionally in a homelike setting with Contact Guard and minimal assistance
- perform simple homemaking tasks with minimal assistance.

The plan is for ADL training, functional mobility, perceptual-motor skills, left upper extremity neuromuscular retraining, and homemaking six times a week for 8 weeks.

Motivational obstacles for Mrs. N. are extreme anxiety, short attention span, easy distractibility, and impulsivity.

The therapist's problem or dilemma was that Mrs. N. was to return home to live with her husband who is partially disabled. The home is two stories, and minimum family support is available.

Safety issues are a large concern, and Mrs N. and her husband are resistant to adaptive equipment, home modifications, and exploration of other living situations.

—*Rhoda Dorfzaun, OTR/L*
—*Susan Pierce, COTA/L*
—*Maura Hinkle, OTR/L, Director of OT*

Answer

Mrs. N. presents a problem to her therapists: Can she return home to live with a partially disabled husband who resists adaptations, modifications, or moving to another domicile so she can perform safely?

Her motivational obstacles have been identified as extreme anxiety, short attention span, easy distractibility, and impulsivity. Motivation is a function of psychological behavior, which can be adversely affected by neurological damage. It is necessary to assess if Mrs. N.'s "nervous" responses as seen in her occupational therapy rehabilitation program are the result of her long-standing emotional problems, which have been intractable, or are neurological ones that can permanently diminish her functional ability. Because organicity distorts thought and can render unrealistic and/or inaccurate the patient's perception of her nuclear problem (and everything else, as well), psychological tests like the Mini Mental Status Exam should be given to assess cognition.

Mrs. N.'s multiple diagnoses affect her functional performance so that she needs assistance in most areas. Let us analyze the diagnoses.

1. Hemorrhagic CVA to right thalamus can compromise her limbic system, interfering with her endocrine balance; her emotional instability; circadian rhythms; and perceptual, sensory and motor abilities. Permanent damage is likely.

2. Macular degeneration causes progressive central vision loss. The CVA could cause left hemianopsia (left field loss). She might not be able to work at midline nor to her left.

3. Hypothyroidism causes decreased energy and may cause weight gain, making transfers and standing activity difficult.

4. Depression and chronic anxiety of a 15-year-plus duration would decrease creativity and render change very difficult. Her recent cerebral insults most likely increase the effect of both her depression and anxiety.

Mrs. N. is a poorly functioning patient, whose medical condition indicates a poor rehabilitation prognosis. I believe that it is unrealistic for her to return home and that she cannot safely assume homemaking responsibilities, especially since the family is resisting adaptations or change.

It appears likely that Mrs. N. will stay in the nursing home. Occupational therapy should discharge her from active treatment and refer her to recreation for music to calm and alleviate anxiety, and to cooking and chat groups. Because of her vision loss, she should be referred to Lighthouse for the Blind for taped or large print books.

—*Jane Sorensen, PhD, OTR/L*

◆   ◆   ◆

ACCEPTING TREATMENT: FAILURE OR LIMITED SUCCESS

An 84-year-old male was admitted to a subacute facility from a rehabilitation hospital. He suffered a left CVA with dense right hemiparesis. Prior to admission, the patient was active and independent in all ADL. Medical information sent with the patient was sketchy. No occupational therapy report was sent, nor neuropsychological information, magnetic resonance imaging (MRI), or computed axial tomography (CAT) scan. The patient presented as aphasic expressively. He was apraxic. The patient also had a gastrostomy tube placed prior to admission to the skilled nursing facility (SNF). Functionally, the patient required maximum assistance in bathing and dressing and maximum assistance with bed mobility. The patient required maximum assistance of two to squat pivot transfer into the wheelchair.

The patient has a supportive family. He has three sons and a wife. The sons all have families of their own. The patient is the patriarch of the family. Former occupations included electrician and professional wrestler. He enjoys watching game shows on television as well as golf. The patient also enjoys spending time with his family as well as with his grandchildren. His wife has difficulty understanding instructions regarding the patient's care even after repeated attempts to explain by the therapists.

The patient's goals are difficult to identify secondary to aphasia and apraxia. He presents with depressed mood and is combative at times. He displays socially inappropriate behaviors such as expectorating phlegm into his hand and expecting staff to clean this for him. He is unmotivated for therapy. An example of this is the patient's ability to doff shoes, TED hose, and shirt. However, he is unwilling to participate in these activities during therapy. One coping strategy presented by the patient is tuning people out when they attempt to engage.

The family expressed that they would like to have their father return home. The patient appears to have good receptive skills and has the ability to follow two-step tasks. Goals have been set for minimum assistance in bathing and dressing. Goals for function have been set for supervised level bed to chair and chair to commode transfers. He is seen by occupational therapy for 1–1 1/2 hours 6 days a week.

The patient's response varies during therapy. At first he would not participate in any ADL tasks. He would only participate in gross motor tasks. At times he would even stop lifting weights and allow them to hit him. Eventually, he did start to participate in upper body ADL. He seems to respond to limit setting and consistent therapy. The therapist at times feels intimidated by the patient because he pulls her hair or squeezes her hand very tightly.

The problem is how to get full cooperation from this man. How firm should one be with limit setting? How do occupational therapists know if family goals and patient goals are consistent?

—*Renee Lundfelt, OTR/L*

Answer

This book emphasizes the therapist's role in creating a positive motivational context for treatment. Many patients are eager to accomplish rehabilitation goals. They work well with almost any therapist. Others require a great deal of a therapist's understanding, care, and strategizing in order to successfully negotiate the rehabilitation process.

This 84-year-old CVA patient serves as a reminder that even the most effective motivational strategies can fail. Working in the same facility with the therapist who submitted this case, I observed her efforts over time. She did a great job. At first she absorbed some physical abuse from this 270-pound man and tolerated significant frustration due to his resistance. His aphasia obviated all but the most rudimentary communication and hampered collaboration, along with exploration and negotiation of treatment obstacles. Family members were not substantially able to help in understanding the patient's wishes or in identifying formerly valued interests.

Nonetheless, the therapist did not retreat. She attempted to talk to the patient about his illness, his losses, and possibilities for the future, although she received little response. She set firm limits on assaultive behaviors, established a daily routine, explained treatment goals and procedures, offered clear instructions, graded task expectations, and provided a lot of verbal rein-

forcement. A course of antidepressant medication was begun, following a psychiatric consult.

The patient did respond initially. His transfer skills and ADL participation improved incrementally, and assaultive behavior diminished. The treatment was a partial and temporary success. Within a month, however, the patient plateaued, and acting-out behavior and resistance resurfaced. Family members failed to learn caregiving skills despite repeated efforts, and skilled services were finally discontinued. The man became a permanent resident in the nursing home, requiring maximum assistance for all activities.

Some therapists might conclude that this patient had poor rehabilitation potential, that treatment failure was a foregone conclusion, and that skilled services should not have been provided. It is true that a relatively poor medical prognosis, unclear hopes, assaultive response to helpers, and poor task performance were detracting factors. However, the patient did have a supportive family who wanted him home. He possessed significant residual physical strength, and he did respond well to a consistent, directive approach. Frequently, a borderline case is worthy of a trial run. People can respond to trouble and to treatment in surprising ways. In this instance, however, a number of factors conspired to defeat the rehabilitation process.

I suspect this patient perceived that he had lost much, and had so little to gain, that his will to try was fleeting and thin. Wants, beliefs, and rewards related to treatment were weak. Given his large size, significant paralysis, and cognitive, perceptual, and communication deficits, the costs of rehabilitation, in contrast, were great. Even if he could return home, given the family's limitations, he may have had little confidence in the care he would receive there. Despite early efforts, the man's helpless anger, confusion, impulsivity, and the agonizing effort to communicate and accomplish even the simplest task prevailed. In the end, the obstacles to sustained motivation and to treatment were just too great. Even a resourceful and determined therapist could not succeed.

This case has been included so that treatment failure can be recognized, accepted, and normalized as a realistic part of occupational therapy practice. As therapists, we have significant responsibilities, authority, and skill; but we do not hold all of the cards. We and our patients can only do our best to play the hands we are dealt.

—Mark S. Rosenfeld, PhD, OTR

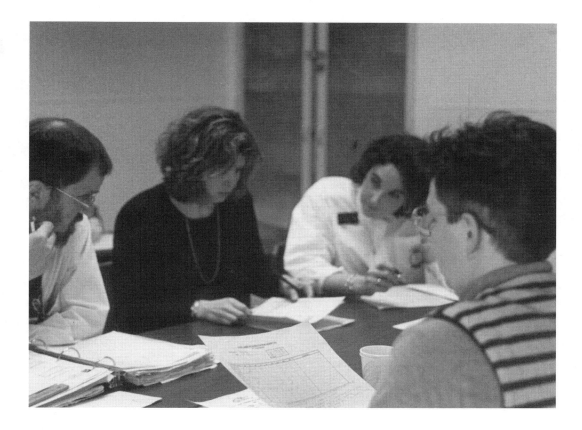

Chapter 4 *Documentation and Reimbursement of Motivational Interventions in Long-Term Care*

Warren F. Dahlin, Jr., MS, OTR/L

We know that our professional survival depends on these two important concepts—documentation and reimbursement. The challenge in writing this chapter was complex. I feared that, given the rate of change of the current health care system and our profession, almost anything I wrote would be useless within a year. Another concern was that incorrect information in this important area could actually lead to increased problems in our profession. I know that the responsibility is great. I know too that when we sit down to document what we have just seen and done with our patients there are great risks. A mistake or omission in our work at this critical point can result in a refusal for reimbursement and an inability to continue to provide desperately needed treatment. Perhaps the most threatening of all possibilities is that what we write or do not write can result in criticism or pain. Few long-term-care providers work or write without fearing censure for poorly done documentation or without facing the conflicting motives of some profit-making, budget-conscious, nonclinician bureaucrat.

It is important to acknowledge the pain associated with documentation and reimbursement. Without doing so, this chapter will not be helpful. If you associate documentation and reimbursement with pain instead of pleasure, it is hard to imagine how your work could be of the highest quality. If documentation can be something that generates feelings of joy, satisfaction, and pride, on the other hand, not only will the quality of your professional life improve, but you will enjoy a new era of improvement and growth as a key player in this changing health care system and society.

Just as the task of documentation engenders discomfort in a majority of therapists, so does the process of defining occupational therapy. However, the one central truth that appears in every discussion or definition of our profession is the *use of activity*. It is a universal truth that occupational therapists appreciate and use activity to promote change, growth, and health. Why is it so hard for us to see the activity of documentation as a *therapeutic activity* for ourselves and our profession? Do we practice what we preach? Is there a way that we could attack the activity of documenting in the chart with the same excitement with which we expect our clients to embark on the therapeutic activities we prescribe?

When I shifted my own consciousness in performing the task of writing the words you are now reading, a major change occurred. I knew this chapter was needed and felt it "should" be done. Quite frankly, there were other things I would rather write about. In fact, this would have been my last choice! I had fears that it wouldn't be helpful, the editor would not like it, that people would find out I was not sure of myself, that rapid change would make this outdated, or that I might provide people with wrong advice.

When I realized that all these feelings were unpleasant and painful, I consciously changed my focus. With determination to transform pain to pleasure, I decided to tackle this chapter with gusto. The moment I became convinced that I could begin writing with the belief that this would be enjoyable, pleasurable, and useful, a major shift did occur. This conscious shift in focus brought instant and profound change. As I sit here, bent over my keyboard, bathed in blue light from my computer screen, I am having fun. I wish you were here and I wish you were feeling as good as I feel right now. I am documenting and it feels good! This is a therapeutic activity. This is occupational therapy. "Physician, heal thyself." This is a great place to start. I cannot wait to try this at work!

At the beginning of this chapter we stressed that documentation is the key

to survival. As I write this I realize the danger of that wrong message. That message instills fear and anxiety. Rather than go back and change it, however, it is more instructive to leave the "error" in the first paragraph as a record of how writing changes and clarifies our cognitive process. In working with a patient in a home evaluation, do we say, "If you don't remove those scatter rugs you're going to fall again and break another hip!" Or instead, do we expect the person to change the environment so that safety, health, and a long-term feeling of well-being permeates his or her existence? Is it not better to give our patients comfortable and supportive messages?

Now let us treat ourselves with the same positive approach. We need to give ourselves and each other active support and encouragement for efforts to improve our documentation. Some of the rewards that will come from this shift in focus will include increased professional effectiveness and continued reimbursement. Better documentation will lead to increased respect for occupational therapy.

WHAT IS WRITING?

Writing is thinking visualized. Once we write something, it becomes more clear. Through writing we improve our cognitive acuity and clinical practice. For many of us, taught in American schools, writing itself is connected with a great deal of pain. Julia Cameron in *The Artist's Way* (1992) suggests that we are victims of our "creative monsters," that people in our past—teachers, parents, supervisors, and others—have sent strong messages to us that our writing is not good. In our profession these creative monsters are everywhere. They may be critical surveyors, supervisors, cost-conscious administrators, or the voices of our old teachers. If left unchecked, these voices become our own and we play our own negative tapes as we write. Silence negative forces and begin to enjoy the writing process. Believe in yourself as much as we believe in the people with whom we work. The following case demonstrates this idea.

Years ago I had a patient, who I will call Mr. Simon, who came to our long-term-care facility for short-term cardiac rehabilitation after a serious quintuple bypass. His blood pressure fluctuated dangerously, and he appeared depressed. In trying to set a climate in which he would be comfortable talking, I told him about a student who said, "Sometimes I feel like crying, but I'm afraid if I started I would never be able to stop." I asked my patient if he ever felt like that.

His response was both interesting and frightening. He said, "No, that's not how it feels. It feels like, if I ever let out the pressure that was in me, I would explode." This was a horrifying metaphor for a post-surgical bypass patient with uncontrolled blood pressure. I asked if he could transform the metaphor to a dam, where he and I could open a series of release valves and gently lower the level of water to an acceptable level in a controlled way. He did not believe it was possible but said he would love it if that could happen,

stating that no one had ever discussed the relationship of his stress level to his cardiac condition.

For the next few days we worked on increasing endurance, conserving energy, managing pain, training in safety, learning to self-monitor, and most important to him, relieving pressure! This domain required the skill of an occupational therapist because it involved a constant monitoring of his medical status and manipulation of vital signs through purposeful activity. The causes of his stress were far too complicated to outline here, but the unresolved grief of the loss of his wife and the family conflict between his children were major sources. He wished he could talk to his wife. I suggested that he put down his thoughts in writing. In effect, I was asking him to document his thoughts and the events of his life. Is that not what documentation asks of all of us? My request had the same effect on him as the task of documentation has on most of us.

His response was immediately negative. He said that he was not very smart (not true according to my observations and his performance) and that he only had a high school diploma. He said he could not write. I asked if there was any time when he ever wrote. He said, "Oh sure, during World War II my wife and I constantly wrote long letters. I still read them sometimes. They give me great pleasure." I asked him how long she had been dead and he said, "Almost 10 years." My response was, "Then don't you think it's about time you wrote her again to catch her up on what's been happening?"

I shall never forget the expression on this man's face when the words sunk in, when he realized how much he would enjoy writing those letters, how much he had to say, how easy, helpful and valuable the activity would be. I wish I could share here some of the hundreds of beautiful pages he wrote. I wish I could be there after his death to watch his children's reactions to his carefully stored record of a beautiful love affair and an admirable life. I wish I could see the results of the admonitions and suggestions that will come after his death through his written records to children who were seldom able to agree or enjoy what they had. He has left his progeny the gift of a lifetime, and through the therapeutic activity of "documentation" he learned to live again. We need that motivation when we chart our work. Writing is thinking visualized.

One of the greatest lessons of this case example is the importance of convincing ourselves that we can write. A phrase taken from the keynote speech and repeated for days during the 1995 Great Southern Conference was "I'm an OT. I can do that!" We need that attitude to accomplish documentation that works.

Taking an example from Mr. Simon, we must ask ourselves if there was ever a time when writing brought us joy, and tap into the feeling of that experience. At the risk of sounding terribly behavioralistic, we must extinguish the pain of the documentation process and replace it with pleasure.

ENJOY DOCUMENTATION?

In preparing this chapter, I interviewed many clinicians and OT directors about its basic premise. When it was suggested that ideally we need to transform the pain of documentation into pleasurable experience, most therapists responded with comments like, "You'll never do that!" Some responded with a smirk and said things like "Yeah, right!" Is this the response we need as a profession?

James Sellers, OTR, Director of Occupational Therapy for New England Sinai Hospital in Stoughton, Massachusetts, was the most positive of all clinicians questioned. His immediate response was to say, "That's very interesting. I don't know if it's possible, but it's a very interesting idea. How could we do that?" Contrast that to the "Yeah, right!" response. His positive response came as no surprise, as he was in the process of transforming his department's documentation to eliminate duplication of effort and decrease time spent writing useless information. "Many people think more is better and that just isn't so," he said with confidence. This is the attitude that will transform our documentation. We must progress!

When Jim asked his staff if they could get rid of one thing in their job, what would it be, the immediate and universal response was "Documentation!" As a fine leader in long-term care, he strives to listen to the needs of his staff and to develop a better way. It is our assumption that, if questioned further, the conscientious therapists of New England Sinai Hospital would not really want to get rid of documentation, but instead would eliminate the pain and discomfort that surrounds the documentation process.

In examining the original *ROTE* manual (1986) that AOTA has used for the past 10 years as the primary vehicle for training occupational therapists who work in long-term care, one is hard pressed to find any reference to documentation or its relationship to reimbursement. We need to encourage and support our professional organizations to explore the issues and skills associated with documentation, and we need to expect that mission to be carried out in a positive and proactive way.

New issues point to changes in documentation that are quite disturbing. Recent flyers in my mailbox advertised new computerized systems that claim to "virtually eliminate the need to document." When so many professionals already maintain open hatred for documentation, this kind of thinking can be very dangerous. Is it in the best interests of our clients and profession to eliminate documentation? Instead we need to create systems in which fine writing reflects both fine thinking and effective work.

It is doubtful that computerized reports will fill readers of those reports with respect and high value for our profession. Documentation tools must be constructed in a careful way to describe a patient's strengths as well as weaknesses. Another issue facing clinicians is the proliferation of checklists and jargon. The managed care gatekeeper is seldom an occupational therapist, and if the gatekeeper does not understand the jargon or know how to read the checklist, services may be denied.

HOW CAN WRITING PRESERVE SERVICES?

I observed a recent case in which the benefits coordinator hundreds of miles away denied an extension of rehabilitation for a 68-year-old man who was a member of a religious order. He had survived a cerebral aneurysm. He had been doing extremely well in occupational therapy using a dowel and washer exercise to increase eye-hand coordination, shoulder extension, and endurance. However, he did not like doing the exercises. The occupational therapist transformed the experience instantly by suggesting that he use the exercise board in the privacy of his room and use it to replace the function of rosary beads (which he was unable to hold and manipulate). The man could not wait to get to his room and worked for hours daily, making major strides.

The refusal to continue reimbursement came as a great surprise to the therapist, who had been documenting remarkable progress. When he explored the issue, the occupational therapist learned that the company's case manager had spoken to the social worker, the neurologist, and the physical therapist after reviewing all their notes. As far as he knew, she had not read the occupational therapist's notes. He called the woman to discuss the situation and found that she had a high school diploma and understood little if any of the discussions or documentation the other professionals had sent. She said she had not read his notes. He observed that she had an Irish name, which increased the probability that she was Catholic, so he took a risk and asked her. She said she was.

The physical therapist explained that when he first saw the patient, the man could only repeat the word "blessing!" and was blind on one side. He remarked that if you could say only one word, this probably was not the worst word to get stuck on. He explained how the washer and dowel board used as a rosary had helped with motivation, speech, endurance, and coordination, "and if you allow me one more month, Miss O'Brien," he stated, "I think occupational therapy will have him healthy enough that he'll be able to say Mass!" He also politely but factually suggested, "If you don't approve the services, I doubt he'll be able to return to his community." This she understood.

The therapist suggested she review the occupational therapy documentation stating the happy facts in clear simple language and the coordinator cheerfully approved the man's stay for rehabilitation for another month. This extension was ample to meet the goal of successful discharge. He now lives in his own apartment at his old religious community and requires only minimal assistance with reading and sending mail. Had the documentation not been prepared in readable form, it is highly probable that he would still be living in a nursing home.

WHAT IS GOOD WRITING?

We have stated that writing is thinking visualized. It is important to consider the purpose of documentation. Of course it is a record, and we have all heard the adage, "If you don't document it, you haven't done it!" and yet, much of the fine work we do is not documented. In the example above, services would not have been extended if the occupational therapist had documented and communicated in the same manner and form as his colleagues. Documentation communicates. Fun and pleasure reside with this communication, and it is here where we can strengthen our skills while supporting our profession.

Think of the work you do every day and ask yourself how important the documentation is. Do you read all of the documentation before walking into the patient's room or visiting the client's home? Is it the written word on which you depend as you work with the client? Of course, what we read about the client is extremely important, and I do not suggest we treat patients without reading the chart. However, in the current practice of occupational therapy, it is useful to consider how much we depend on oral communication.

We often make decisions and share information at patient care meetings, at chance discussions as family and visitors come and go, and as we get last-minute observations from the charge nurse when we come on the ward. Now think, for a moment, about the nature of those discussions. Are they all negative? Are they all unpleasant? Reflecting on many of those discussions, we see the joys of our labor. We share the wonderful stories of something that worked, or we ponder a critical issue that explains what happened or did not happen. We question our assumptions and receive instant feedback about our interactions and our methods. We look for the pieces that work. We learn about the people with whom we work. These times of speaking about our clients and our work often stand out as special times in long-term care. In this clinical specialty area, most successful clinicians find great joy in small gains. We can and often must accept the pain of repeated failures. In long-term care, the most difficult and sometimes abandoned individuals whom we successfully treat often become our greatest triumphs. These events carry us through the day. Where can we read about them?

It is certain that every person who wrote and sent a case study for this book is better off as a clinician and a person because they made the effort. It is a good bet that everyone who wrote about those cases better understands their role. It is also highly probable that during and after writing, the authors discussed their related thoughts with their friends and colleagues and, I hope, with the patients themselves. If these assumptions are true, it is also safe to assume that when those discussions took place, they were more instructive and productive because of the writing that preceded the discussion. So let us write about our victories!

THE CHALLENGE

Part of the difficulty of documentation exists because frequently the chart does not fully reflect what happens during the treatment. Central to this discussion is the fact that the wonderful motivation strategies that we use are the very items we leave out of the documentation. If we record these, not only will the task of writing be more pleasurable but we also will educate nonoccupational therapists of the true value of our profession.

Therapists have discussed the challenge of documentation as a tool to ensure that services are not discontinued. This is a particularly important issue in long-term care because gains are often small in a system that requires ongoing, marked progress. Thus, the dilemma. How do we document without killing the patient's chances? This takes on new meaning as we consider outcomes.

In *Nationally Speaking*, published in *AJOT* (1996), Mary Foto stressed the importance of conducting outcomes research. It is essential to consider this importance when making a shift toward more effective documentation, since our future seems to depend on outcomes and provides us with a marvelous opportunity for improvement. Foto suggests that our profession demonstrates both efficacy and cost-effectiveness. Do our current documentation processes reflect these factors in long-term care? Unlike goals, outcomes speak to the value of the service. Do our notes do that?

In her important call to action, Foto outlined questions that focus on four key service delivery measurements. Consider these issues as we explore more effective methods of recording our worth.

Effectiveness

- Of the array of assessment procedures available for each diagnostic group, which most accurately and consistently identify and define that group's impairments and disabilities?

◆ Of the array of treatment procedures available, which produce the expected increase in functional status most consistently?

Efficiency

Of the array of assessment procedures available for each diagnostic group, which

◆ take the least amount of time to accurately identify and define the impairments and disabilities of that group?

◆ are absolutely necessary to identify and define that group's impairments and disabilities?

Of the treatment procedures available, which

◆ take the least amount of time to produce the expected increase in functional status?

◆ are absolutely necessary to produce the expected increase in functional status?

◆ produce an increase in functional status that is maintained across time without further therapeutic intervention?

Of the assessment and treatment procedures, which has the highest correlation with the best outcomes?

Quality

Quality is defined in terms of the provision of clinical services that are the most

◆ appropriate—assessment and treatment procedures that are the most specific and effective to the needs of a specific diagnostic group.

◆ effective—assessment and treatment procedures that have the highest correlation with the greatest functional gains.

◆ efficient—assessment and treatment procedures that have the highest correlation with both the greatest functional gains and the least frequency, intensity, and duration of treatment as well as the greatest durability.

Value

In terms of value, do the gains in function that result from our clinical services also result in

◆ greater ability of the persons of a diagnostic group to participate in life?

◆ high patient satisfaction?

◆ holding down of overall costs (i.e., prevent illness or conditions for which patients are at higher risk due to their impairments or disabilities, contribute to reducing length of stay, prevent rehospitalization, and reduce collateral caregiver costs)?

Referring back to the case of the priest, with respect to effectiveness, efficiency, quality, and values, it is not only possible but enjoyable to speak in these terms.

In terms of effectiveness, occupational therapy worked well with the patient while other disciplines failed to motivate the man. The challenge was to document this in a way that did not lead to refusal of other services. The occupational therapist wrote, "Increased motivation in occupational therapy led to increased participation in other services." Striving to see the whole picture when we write makes things far more interesting and pleasurable. (If a person comes to my facility with an occupational therapy referral stating "no occupational therapy needed," it obviously makes it more difficult to justify necessary treatment.)

Efficiency becomes obvious when we consider this individual being guided and coaxed through a therapeutic process, who is suddenly transformed through occupational therapy and who now takes over his own treatment. This smacks of efficiency! Again, it is fun to write about.

Quality includes appropriateness of services, diagnostic tools, and therapeutic decisions. How appropriate is it to have a priest repeatedly reaching to place little washers on a wooden stick? How understandable we become as therapists when we translate our tasks into plain talk that addresses individual's actual needs and desires. Because we deal with function and easily understood tasks and needs, occupational therapy is actually one of the easiest services to document. Efficiency and effectiveness are both measures of quality. For example, the therapist wrote, "Patient refuses to participate in strengthening and visual tracking exercises." The plan stated, "Transform equipment and modify procedures so that the patient (a priest) can pray while doing the exercises."

Values become our strongest tool, and it is here where the pleasure and pride surge. The continued services for the priest were approved more for their value than for any other reason. The documentation indicated that with continued treatment the priest would be able to return as a participating member of his community, and that the services would lead to savings. One month of rehabilitation and return home is an insignificant cost compared with spending the rest of one's life in a nursing home.

In addition to Mary Foto's well-structured advice, every occupational therapist would be better served by rereading "Value Laden Beliefs and Principles for Rehabilitation" (Wright, 1981). As budgets are cut and the very profession of occupational therapy is in danger of being diluted and eliminated, arguing from a point of value-laden beliefs becomes a strong force. Sixty years ago, Britain insisted that subjects of India could neither spin cloth nor make salt. Mahatma Gandhi managed to topple the empire with his homemade spinning wheel and a hand full of salt he gathered while facing a loaded rifle. He triumphed because his values were based on truth. However, it was the truth and the exposure of oppression that Gandhi saw as the real force. This, in itself, is a strong, value-laden belief, and it is important for occupational therapists today. Cutting vital services to save money is as morally repugnant as preventing people of India from making their own cloth. To write clearly about our effective motivational strategies and their value is to reflect our value and worth in a way that would make denial of services far more difficult.

As therapists, we have our own values that are not only worth examining but also worth including in our notes. In Wright's (1981, p. 266) article, the first value states, "The patient needs respect and encouragement." It is important not only to think about this value but also to wonder how we might include this in our documentation. Again, this is the real power (and fun) of writing. Another of Wright's values states that the patient will be part of the planning process. Our desire to continue services is much stronger when our work and notes reflect this important value.

IMPORTANT TIPS FOR OCCUPATIONAL THERAPISTS WHO DOCUMENT

I use techniques outlined in *Writing the Natural Way* (Rico, 1983), which suggests placing a central idea in the middle of a page. Around this idea, other ideas sprout that are connected by lines and circled. From them, lines are drawn and other ideas are written and circled. Before long, a page could be filled with

key words that the author suggests are clustered in patterns established by the "design mind" of the writer.

My writing and the writing of my students has vastly improved after using this method. In the spirit of Mary Foto's aforementioned suggestions, this idea could be modified. The patient's initials or number could be written in the middle of the page and toward each corner, the words efficiency, quality, effectiveness, and values. As we jot down a single word or phrases in relationship to these important outcome measures, our work would take on new meaning (see example below). This is not to be seen by anyone but the therapist and is only a technique used to promote clearer thinking. However, like all good documentation, it can be used as a therapeutic modality as well since it helps the writer to perceive and organize critical facts that should be included in the

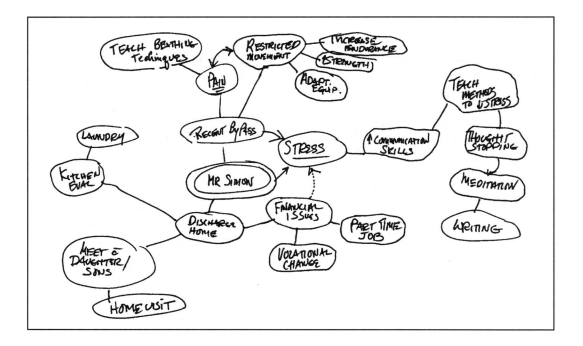

evaluation summary, treatment plan, and progress note.

Another fascinating design that helps to examine and map what is happening in therapy may be found by using the four quadrants suggested by Ken Wilber in *A Brief History of Everything* (1996). He presents an astonishingly simple, clear method of analyzing information using a four-quadrant grid including Interior-Individual (sensory/cultural), Exterior-Individual (biological/observable), Interior-Collective (cultural), and Exterior-Collective (social). This groundbreaking work is essential for understanding and documenting occupational therapy.

ALL DOCUMENTATION MAY NOT BE WRITING

A picture is worth a thousand words! This saves considerable time and permits clearer communication.

If we accept the assumption that documentation is communication, then we might expand our traditional view and use some of the wonderful skills we possess. One of these skills may be drawing. Many occupational therapists draw very well. If you do not, then obtain and use *Drawing With the Right Side of Your Brain* by Betty Edwards (1989). Often, a simple line drawing showing the present condition and the expected condition can be extremely effective. In developing the Therapy Carrot Finger Orthosis™ (see example below), it was important for me to get the message across as quickly as possible because it was a new treatment procedure and device for working with people with severe hand contractures. Traditionally, it has been difficult to get reimbursement for these "chronic" problems, yet national surveys have increased their focus on hand care in

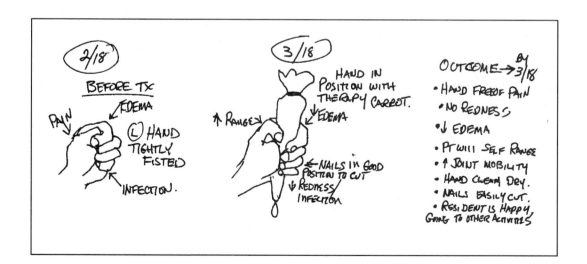

long-term-care facilities. Documentation was key in facilitating the use of this new method and product. A simple line drawing of a condition before and after, or a picture of a piece of equipment in the correct position instead of the wrong position, can create interest, curiosity, respect, and understanding in the people who use the chart as a guide to providing or paying for the service.

These line drawings take up very little space and really draw attention to the message we want to get across. Did they catch your eye as you looked through this book? On page three of a standard discharge referral, a simple, well-done line drawing will definitely catch the attention of the home-health personnel. These people are often critical to making the discharge plan an effective reality. Documentation is a way to impress on others the effectiveness of occupational therapy.

SUMMARY

Documentation may not equate with pleasure—yet. By using some of the hints in this chapter, you and your patients may have some pleasant surprises. Consider writing as a therapeutic activity to heal an ailing health care system. Believe in the process of occupational therapy. Structure documentation so that it reflects outcomes and is easily understandable, free of jargon, and reflective of the strengths of our clients and our profession. Remember that motivational strategies are effective and pleasurable both to do and to write about. Let us ensure that those responsible for approving payment for our

continued service get to read about and understand the wonderful motivational strategies this book suggests.

Examine the four key service delivery measures of efficiency, effectiveness, quality, and value, and learn to speak to these issues in your notes. Create work that reflects joy and strong, value-laden beliefs. Employ creative methods like free writing and drawing to encourage others to read our notes and thereby appreciate the wonderful art and science of occupational therapy.

REFERENCES

Cameron, J. (1992). *The artist's way: A spiritual path to higher creativity.* New York: Tarcher/Putnam.

Edwards, B. (1989). *Drawing with the right side of your brain.* New York: Jeremy Tarcher.

Foto, M. (1996). Outcome studies: The what, why, how, and when. *American Journal of Occupational Therapy, 58,* 87-88.

Rico, G.L. (1983). *Writing the natural way.* New York: Tarcher/Putnam.

ROTE. (1986). Bethesda, MD. American Occupational Therapy Association.

Wilber, K. (1996). *A brief history of everything.* Boston: Shambhala Publications.

Wright, B.A. (1981). Value laden beliefs and principles for rehabilitation. *Rehabiliation Literature, 42,* 266-268.

SUGGESTED READINGS

Allen, P.B. (1995). *Art is a way of knowing.* Boston: Shambhala Publications.

Dahlin, W. (1994). *Working with the dififcult client and staff.* Presentation at Second Annual Geriatric Rehabilitation Conference, Cambridge, MA.

Dahlin, W. (1995). Keynote address. Address presented at The Great Southern, Little Rock, AR.

Dahlin, W. (1996). Treatment and reimbursement of upper extremity contracture care in long term care settings. *Common problems, useful solutions.* Dedham, MA: AliMed, Inc.

Edwards, B. (1989). *Drawing with the right side of the brain.* New York: Jeremy Tarcher.

Elbow, P. (1973). *Writing without teachers.* London: Oxford University Press.

Hagon, C. (1994). *Managing cost and quality in brain injury rehabilitation: Understanding the case manager's perspective.* Paper presented at San Pedro Peninsula Hospital, San Pedro, CA.

Editor's Suggestion:

To receive reimbursement for holistic treatment interventions, it is important to include the following items in occupational therapy documentation:

- **Describe occupations used and their strategic purpose** (insurers will not understand the value of occupational interventions unless we teach them).

- **Cite specific progress toward functional goals in areas of ADL, productivity (work/study), and leisure** (a functional life includes a balance in these areas).

- **Explain therapeutic strategies used to clarify goals and increase motivation** (*reflecting* and *planning* are important along with *doing* in the occupational therapy process. Psychosocial and cognitive obstacles must be overcome along with physical ones for successful adaptation to occur).

A progress note illustration from the treatment of a bedridden, depressed woman with severe rheumatoid arthritis:

Phyllis attended OT treatment 3x this week, after refusing all sessions previous week. She transferred Mod Assist and was out of bed for 1–2 hours each of the 3 days. Pt planted indoor bulbs. This occupation is related to pt's report of a life-long leisure interest in gardening, and motivated the pt to be OOB for the first time in a week. Pt planted 12 bulbs in 4 pots, requiring Mod Assist to dig with tool. She demonstrated 75° shoulder flexion and good BL coordination to plant, cover, and water bulbs. Pt followed instructions for joint protection and energy conservation and was able to recall instructions at end of each session. Cognitive endurance and sitting tolerance increased from 1 to 2 hours by end of week. Mood brightened as evidenced by pt's smiles, positive self-statements re performance, and gracious response to compliments on sprouting bulbs from nursing staff and residents. Phyllis has requested assistance to be OOB each day next week to water and tend bulbs. Recommend continued use of horticultural occupations as part of program to improve mobility, UE, and safety skills in performance of self-care, productivity, and leisure tasks.

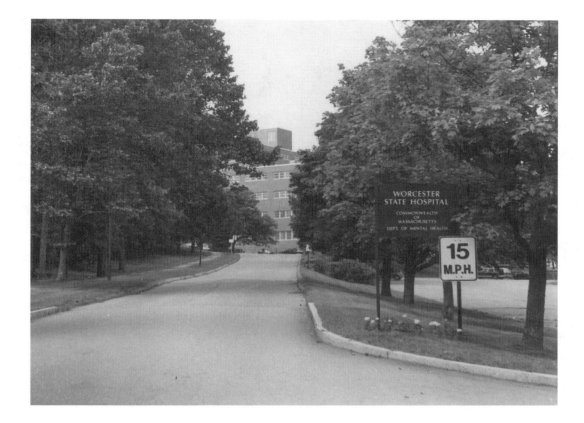

Chapter **5** *Motivational Strategies in Geropsychiatry*

Janice Hengel, MGA, MS, OTR/L

Geropsychiatry is often thought of as a narrow sub-specialty within the medical specialty of psychiatry. In reality, the geropsychiatric population is broad, diverse, and complex. The term *geriatric*, which refers to the aged, encompasses all segments of society. The term *psychiatric*, which refers to mental, emotional, or behavioral disorders, also encompasses all segments of society and is interwoven with medical, economic, and social problems (Clark, 1995; Schaft & Randolph, 1994). A portion of the geropsychiatric population includes the chronic mentally ill who have grown old in institutions with only brief periods spent in the community. Another portion had no history of psychiatric disorders until late in life, when multiple losses compounded the difficulty of coping with everyday stressors. Two psychiatric disorders that are particularly associated with the elderly are depression and organic brain syndrome (Cohen, 1982; Gaitz & Varner, 1982; Reisberg & Ferris, 1982). These disorders can affect anyone, whether in an institution or the community and with or without a history of mental illness.

Creating a positive vision of one's life based on past experiences, beliefs, and values, and perceiving the possibility for continuity of that vision into the future, is a powerful motivator and our greatest challenge. The concept of quality of life is highly personal and dependent on individual and cultural values. Issues of functional independence, autonomy, and control, and issues of interdependence and sense of community, have a subjective meaning and must be personally defined as a part of one's vision (Clark, 1995). The process of occupational therapy uses meaningful activity to define these issues and create a positive vision of the future. As an occupational therapist, my goal is to help each patient create and realize his or her own vision and, thus, discover that which has meaning and is motivating in his or her life.

CASE STUDIES

Mary Ellen

Mary Ellen is 72 years old. She was diagnosed with schizophrenia in her late teens and has lived in a state psychiatric institution almost continuously for the past 50 years. She demonstrated institutional behaviors that made it difficult for her to be discharged to another setting. One such behavior that had particularly annoyed staff and visitors occurred when she would wait by the door for someone to enter the unit. She typically would barrage them with questions, follow them, and, in general, annoy and pester them. For this behavior she received needed attention, but it was usually negative and even punitive. She was frequently told to go sit down and leave people alone. Programs that she had attended to develop social and interpersonal skills did not make a difference in these institutional behaviors.

Because Mary Ellen had behaved this way for so long, it was generally accepted that nothing could be done except for her to learn to leave people alone. Consequently, the staff focused on controlling this behavior rather than changing it, which led to conflict with Mary Ellen, reinforcing her role as a patient with little control over her own life.

A group of occupational therapy students were assigned to Mary Ellen's unit to take a needed, fresh look at what could be done to improve the quality of life and discharge potential for these patients. In Mary Ellen's case, they decided to change this negative behavior into a positive one by making her the unit "greeter" to welcome people as they came onto the unit. This role prescribed behaviors that were already present in the patient's repertoire and did not require new learning. It was a role that was valued by others and viewed as helpful rather than annoying. Her greeting behavior became a source of

positive rather than negative feedback. Mary Ellen's role shifted from that of being exclusively a patient to that of being the unit greeter, which supported her sense of self-worth, autonomy, and control. She performed this role eagerly and well, even when she was transferred to another setting.

Julie

Two years prior to her hospitalization for depression, Julie had experienced a series of losses that led to her attempted suicide. She was a 60-year-old woman with a history of depression dating back 30 years but who was, nonetheless, able to complete graduate school, hold responsible positions at work, and support herself independently. She owned her own home, was unmarried, and had no children. Julie had lived with a significant other for many years. Then she was diagnosed with a progressive neuromuscular disease and experienced a decline in functioning leading to forced retirement; and her significant other died suddenly. Once in the hospital, she became more hopeless and withdrawn when confronted with the possibility of not being able to return to her home. Her economic independence was threatened as a result of her medical bills and the prospect of the ongoing need for nursing home care. Her life had spiraled out of control.

With the intention of engaging her in the treatment process, her treatment team recommended that she participate in the library and creative writing programs. They hoped these activities would renew old interests and stimulate her cognitively. She refused to participate. This was understandable considering that Julie valued her role as an independent and contributing member of society. Now that her independence had been lost, or so she perceived, she could not envision a life for herself that had meaning. There was no reason to pursue old interests under her new, painful circumstances.

Julie did agree to an assessment of her current level of functioning relative to her self-care and maintenance skills. Ultimately, she was challenged cognitively to participate in modifying her environment to increase her level of independence and sense of control over her own life. As the return to her home became a possibility, her efforts were focused on discharge and putting the pieces of her life back in place in a slightly different way. The library and creative writing programs could now be evaluated by her to determine whether they were relevant parts of her future life. Along with other programs and services, they had become tools for realizing her vision.

In both cases, it was necessary to look at the treatment environment to examine how to maximize the individual's performance. Fidler (1995) contends that an environment that ensures elements including autonomy, individuality, and consensual validation fosters a lifestyle that has meaning. In Mary Ellen's case, the students had to look at the behavior from her perspective. By waiting at the door, she was asserting herself in an effort to get the attention of others. The problem was that this behavior led to negative consequences that reinforced her dependent patient

role, which was inconsistent with asserting her autonomy and individuality and establishing reciprocal relationships with others. Further complicating the issue were the facts that she had spent most of her life as a patient and that she would continue to need care after discharge as a patient into another setting. Mary Ellen needed a role within the context of being a patient that had meaning and would improve her quality of life. The unit greeter was such a role because it was valued within the context of the institution, was not shared by other patients, was initiated as she chose, and elicited feedback that verified her contribution.

In Julie's case, timing was everything. She had lost the sense of control over her own life. She perceived that what once had meaning, her independent lifestyle, was no longer possible. Independence was symbolic of control. Through the objective evaluation of her current level of functioning by the occupational therapist, she was able to verify her own perceptions about what she could and could not do relative to living independently. In this way she resumed control over her own life. Participating in other activities helped her to further validate what her skills were, to reconceptualize and reconstruct her lifestyle, and to take control of her future.

REFERENCES

Clark, P. (1995). Quality of life, values, and teamwork in geriatric care: Do we communicate what we mean? *The Gerontologist, 35*, 402–411.

Cohen, G. (1982). The older person, the older patient, and the mental health system. *Hospital and Community Psychiatry, 33*, 101–104.

Fidler, G. (1995). Life-style performance: From profile to conceptual model. *American Journal of Occupational Therapy, 50,* 139–147.

Gaitz, C., & Varner, R. (1982). Principles of mental health care for elderly patients. *Hospital and Community Psychiatry, 33,* 127–133.

Reisberg, B., & Ferris, S. (1982). Diagnosis and assessment of the older patient. *Hospital and Community Psychiatry, 33,* 104–110.

Schaft, G., & Randolph, F. (1994). Innovative community based services for older persons with mental illness. Rockville, MD: Center for Mental Health Services.

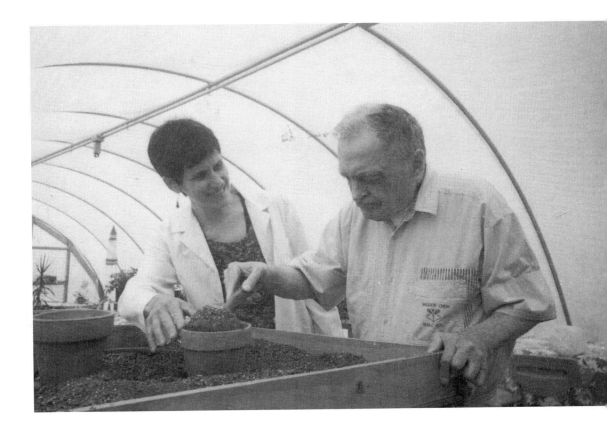

6 *Motivational Strategies for the Older Person with Developmental Disabilities*

Kim Watkins, BS, OTR/L and Susan K. Weiner, OTR/L, MPH

The elderly developmentally disabled population creates a unique challenge to those involved in providing services. An elderly person with developmental disabilities faces many of the changes and losses that any elderly person faces. Advancing medical technology has significantly improved the quality and number of years of life of those with developmental disabilities. In addition, major legislative and social changes have affected habilitative services and the social role people with developmental disabilities play in our community. Services focus on the person's needs and desires rather than on the systems available. By focusing on the person, we support a valued lifestyle and facilitate the contribution of each person in community life. Elderly developmentally disabled persons struggle with the significant challenge of maintaining as much independence as possible and defining their social roles in communities still struggling with the inclusion of those with a developmental disability. Not long ago, people over 55 years of age with developmental disabilities lived almost exclusively in state institutions, in nursing homes, or at home with aging parents. The person who remained at home was frequently placed in a state institution or nursing home when caregivers could no longer care for him or her. Today, the demography of where older people with developmental disabilities live approaches the distribution of the average elderly population (Jacobson, Sutton, & Janicki, 1985).

People who receive services have intermittent to pervasive developmental needs. Many of these individuals have a secondary diagnosis such as cerebral palsy, chronic or childhood psychiatric syndromes, or a medical involvement. They live in a variety of residences including living on their own, housing for the elderly, private homes with other family members, group homes, staffed apartments or large residential units. Some individuals may not need occupational therapy services, others receive occasional consultative service, while others participate in weekly or daily direct therapy. Occupational therapists provide assessment, treatment, or consultation in homes, work settings, or retirement programs, depending on the person's individual needs.

Motivating the individual with developmental disabilities to participate in occupational therapy begins during the assessment of the individual's needs. In addition to evaluating physical status and functional capabilities, it is important to engage the person in assessing what is important to him or her and his or her individual concerns. This information is obtained through interview, good observation of the person's abilities, and the activities the person chooses to do. Often it is helpful to review how the individual spends his or her time and those roles he or she considers important.

Assessments usually occur in the setting in which the concerns or problems arise so that the therapist can take advantage of contextual cues. Assessing the person in his or her work, retirement, or residence often provides critical information as to how that person is actually functioning. First, the individual is usually more comfortable in a familiar setting. Second, the therapist may be able to observe other problem areas.

The following case illustrates the importance of understanding a patient's needs and goals in designing successful occupational therapy treatment.

For many years Joe provided janitorial services for the local air force base. Following the closing of that base, a change in his home of 10 years, and a significant reduction in vision from a retinopathy, Joe began to exhibit signs of depression. He became increasingly isolated and needed much encouragement to complete self-care activities. Joe was referred to occupational therapy

to improve adaptive strategies and participation in activities of daily living, improve mobility, and provide recommendations for retirement activities. Throughout the occupational therapy assessment, Joe expressed his sense of loss by repeatedly asking to go back to work. Therefore, the occupational therapist recommended volunteer janitorial activities at a local senior citizens' center. To achieve his goal, Joe helped develop short-term goals to independently travel in familiar spaces and increase his overall physical condition. He wanted to be able to lift wastebaskets and chairs, which were to be part of his duties at the senior center. In addition, Joe needed to complete his morning routine of bathing, dressing, and eating breakfast so he could get to his day program on time. After Joe joined an exercise group and individual therapy, he began talking about how much he missed his work. He was able to express his loss in a supportive setting while also developing a new social network.

Common occupational therapy treatment modalities for developmentally disabled clients include a variety of services:

- Dysphagia intervention
- Activities of daily living training
- Sensorimotor activities
- Balance, endurance, and strengthening exercises
- Adaptation of the environment to enhance safety
- Vocational skills training
- Development of adaptive strategies for diminishing sensory systems

◆ Endurance and strengthening activities

◆ Adaptive equipment assessment and training.

A person's social and physical environment can significantly influence his or her motivation to participate in therapy to achieve treatment goals. During treatment, familiarity appears to significantly enhance participation and meaning of the treatment activity. Whenever possible, familiar personal possessions, memorabilia, songs, and pictures are used. In addition, it is critical to organize the environment and structure the activities to compensate for sensory and motor deficits. Using simple, colorful visual cues to mark entrances and exits or the location of an activity, limiting auditory distractions, and using natural opportunities for reality orientation help reduce confusion. If low vision is a concern, floors and walls should be different colors to establish borders, and brightly colored objects should be used to facilitate learning.

A common problem arising with aging is the deterioration of activities of daily living skills. Motivating the older person with developmental disabilities to participate in self-care and independent living skills may take a variety of strategies. A history of being assisted by or dependent on caregivers and diminished understanding of the need to perform activities of daily living may hamper the individual's motivation to participate in treatment. Following a thorough assessment of individual needs, the therapist first creates a safe environment. This may mean limiting stimulation to

decrease confusion, providing adaptive equipment, and developing a therapeutic relationship. Next, the therapist works with the person to develop and perform activities that are meaningful, interest the person, are measurable, and lead to the individual's and therapist's desired outcome. For the person who is nonverbal or has difficulty either comprehending or expressing his or her goals or concerns, it is helpful to develop treatment modalities based on the individual's means of expressing his or her approval or disapproval. The therapist can also attempt to gather a history of preferred activities, routines, likes, and dislikes from chart review and discussion with caregivers and family members. When historical data and communication are limited, the therapist must rely on good observation skills and trial and error.

People with developmental disabilities often experience delays or deficits in swallowing abilities. Some factors that contribute to this are an increase in central nervous system dysfunction and long-term psychotropic medication use. Oral-motor and swallowing skills decline with age and can be pronounced in persons with developmental disabilities. Risk factors for safe eating may increase with persons who are edentulous, who eat rapidly, or who put large portions in their mouths. A thorough evaluation may include history; assessment of oral-motor structures and functions; observation; and a video fluoroscopic study to show any of the above problems as well as pooling of food in pockets in the throat, the valleculae, and pyriform sinuses, and aspiration of food or liquids into the lungs. After an evaluation is conducted, a treatment plan including a carefully structured dining program usually is effective. Occasionally problems may be so severe that nonoral feedings are introduced. Positioning, food texture, liquid consistency, amount, and pace in a calm and pleasant environment are critical factors in setting up a safe, successful dining program.

A person who needs to accept a change in food texture may benefit from participating in the preparation of the food or from being offered choices of foods that are safe to eat. When an occupational therapy assessment and video fluoroscopy indicated that Mikhail needed a ground-food consistency, for example, the occupational therapist helped texturize his meal and add some condiments from Mikhail's native country, Russia. This significantly facilitated his acceptance of softer foods.

The elderly person with developmental disabilities needs to practice his or her skills in a safe environment and as they naturally occur. Like any occupational therapy client to be motivated for treatment, individuals with developmental disabilities need options or choices in the treatment plan, an understanding of the desired outcome of the activity, and a sense of control and competence in the skill.

SUGGESTED READINGS

Anderson, D., Lakin, K., Bruininks, R., & Hill, B. (1987). *A national study of residential and support services for elderly persons with mental retardation* (Report No. 22). Minneapolis, MN: University of Minnesota, Department of Educational Psychology.

Bruininks, R., Meyers, C., Sigford, B., & Lakin, C. (Eds.). (1981). Deinstitutionalization and community adjustment of mentally retarded people. In *Compendium of annual conference.* (Monograph 4). Washington, DC: American Association for Mental Retardation.

Crepeau, E. (1986). *Activity programming for the elderly.* Boston: Little Brown.

Jacobson, J., Sutton, M., & Janicki, M. (1985). Demography and characteristics of aging and aged mentally retarded persons. In M.P. Janicki & H.M. Wisniewski (Eds.), *Aging and developmental disabilities, Issues and approaches* (pp. 115–143). Baltimore: Paul H. Brookes.

Keller, M.J. (Ed.). (1991). *Activities with developmentally disabled elderly and older adults.* New York: The Haworth Press.

Seltzer, M., & Krauss, M. (1987). Aging and mental retardation. In *Compendium of annual conference.* (Monograph 9). Washington, DC: American Association for Mental Retardation.

Taira, E. (Ed.). (1991). *The mentally impaired elderly.* Binghamton, NY: The Haworth Press.

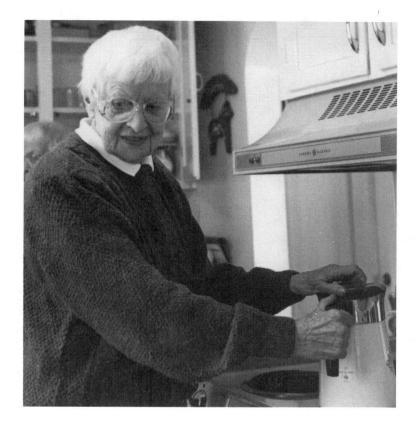

Chapter **7** *Home Health Occupational Therapy: Sink or Swim!*

Vickie Patterson, OTR

The provision of health care delivery in the home can be documented as far back as 1796. Laymen provided care to the sick and elderly at the Boston Dispensary. (The earliest reference to the use of occupational therapy services occurred in the *American Journal of Public Health* in February 1949 [AOTA, 1994].) Reimbursement from Medicare for occupational therapy services in the home began with the Omnibus Reconciliation Act of 1980 (Steinhauer, 1995). This law went into effect in 1981 and, as a result, occupational therapy service provision in the home has grown to become a very integral part of the total picture in the home-health arena.

The very core of the practice of occupational therapy is holistic. We are taught in our schools to consider psychological as well as physical factors when assessing and designing a care plan. Our undergraduate education provides us with a clinical affiliation in psychiatry. We are educated in abnormal psychology and the psychodynamics of groups and families. In no other practice setting is this education more useful than in home health. In the hospital setting, we barely see families. If we make special arrangements to stay "after hours," perhaps we can conduct a brief training session on transfers. Or, perhaps we can conduct an education session regarding the therapeutic necessity of "allowing" the patient to practice the dressing skills or the energy conservation techniques taught. In the rehabilitation setting, family interaction is a little more accessible. A "home evaluation" visit is often performed to assess architectural barriers and equipment needs. Home exercise programs are designed for the purpose of providing the patient and family with a list of the appropriate exercises and activities that should be continued at home just as they were in the rehabilitation center. The outpatient center often provides opportunities for the occupational therapist to assess more closely problems the patient encounters in the home and community. The pitfalls, problems, and realities of dealing with, adapting to, and compensating for an illness or disability become very evident when the patient returns home and is living and functioning in his or her environment. The patient is now better able to give more accurate feedback regarding the realities of adaptation. However, communication is secondhand, at best. The feedback from the patient to the therapist is only as good as the patient's ability to assess his or her own dysfunction. The therapist must still do much trial and error guesswork in offering solutions to problems encountered in the home and community environments. When a suggestion is made regarding a solution for a problem, the patient must go home to "try out" the solution and bring the result back into the outpatient clinic 2 or 3 days later. This method certainly delays successful functional outcomes.

The delivery of occupational therapy in the home-health setting is dramatically different. In home-health occupational therapy, assessments are immediate and problems are obvious. Architectural barriers are stumbled over and family members are present. Most times, an assessment that would have taken 15 minutes of questioning in the rehabilitation center or outpatient clinic is immediate as you enter the home. Family and cultural priority questions are answered, many times, on the front porch, or over the telephone as the therapist calls to schedule the first appointment. The condition of the home, the hygiene of the patient, and the presence or absence of family members can all be answers to questions. These answers can help guide the direction of the treatment plan established by the occupational therapist. The answers can also provide clues for use of possible motivational strategies for the geriatric patient. The therapist may often hear statements

such as, "You can't come too early! We don't get up till 9:00" or "You have to come after my stories are finished." These two statements can provide insight into the family lifestyle and culture, thus giving further direction regarding family priorities. If goal setting is not consistent with patient and family culture, lifestyles, and priorities, then the treatment plan is set up for failure before the therapist even begins.

Another issue affecting motivational strategies concerns the physical and mental health of the person in the role of the patient's caregiver. Many times the patient's caregiver is elderly and has multiple medical problems of his or her own. Home-health therapists are often met at the front door by the harried, over-stressed spouse with many complaints and questions. This situation may leave the therapist wondering who is the actual "patient." In order for treatment outcomes to be successful, the treatment plan designed in the home must take into consideration the needs of all the family members. If the patient's caregiver has medical problems, compliance with the home program is greatly improved if exercises and activities are designed so the patient can accomplish them independently. In this case, assigning exercises that require the participation of the caregiver is a setup for failure. Caregivers exhibiting signs of emotional and physical stress may benefit from attention from the therapist to address those needs. Acknowledging the situation and giving the caregiver "permission" to feel anger and resentment can be helpful in using motivational strategies later in the treatment process. Angry and resentful feelings on the part of the caregiver may also produce guilt; "after all, the patient is sick and can't help it." All these feelings and the resulting behavior and dynamics are often counterproductive to motivational intervention. Unless identified and addressed by the occupational therapist, all these issues will multiply, leading to a dysfunctional therapeutic environment.

Another aspect of concern when seeking to provide motivational techniques involves premorbid ethnic, family, and community roles of the patient. A role shift is often perceived as more disabling than the disability itself. The shift in one member's family role often provides a major stress on the entire family, especially if the ethnic family roles are very historical and deeply entrenched in the traditional culture. For example, the Oriental and Hispanic cultures both have a very strong definition of family. These cultures tend to be fairly closed to "outsiders," choosing to handle the family problems internally. As a result, these families do not actively seek outside help. The male of the family is typically in a position of power and authority. If his disability leaves him with residual difficulty in performing his activities of daily living (ADL), the family tends to provide this "service" for him. Success in training the patient in compensatory techniques for ADL deficits can be a major challenge for the therapist if the family is motivated to continue operating within the traditional ethnic behaviors. In these cases, motivational strategies must be very creative to allow successful outcomes. Additional

convolutions in motivation exist when the occupational therapist and the patient are of the same ethnic background. For example, the female Oriental occupational therapist providing service to a male Oriental patient can be a detrimental factor if she uses her role in the traditional sense. If she uses her ethnic background as a common bond and, at the same time, downplays her "female" role, chances of success in motivating the patient are likely to improve.

Behavioral shifts in family roles should not be discounted as trivial by the occupational therapist. Family roles serve needs for us as individuals and the shifting of these roles often results in unmet emotional or psychological needs. The homemaker who has always been responsible for the family checkbook and must now give up that responsibility due to her disability may feel depressed, useless, and out of control. These feelings can lead to great difficulties with motivation. The astute, creative occupational therapist can use these implied needs as part of the motivation process by planning treatment activities to accomplish steps toward the goal of independent check writing. In addition to the stress the patient experiences in relinquishing activities, the caregiver is often thrust into the position of taking over the particular activity previously belonging to the patient. The result is often feelings of fear, resentment, and anger from the caregiver as a result of suddenly having to take over the physical care of the patient and also the household duties the patient had to give up because of the disability or illness.

Motivational strategies in cases like these can center around enlisting help from the caregiver to facilitate activities that would lead to patient independence. Obviously, for caregiver and patient motivation to exist, the occupational therapist needs to be sure patient, caregiver, and therapist goals are consistent.

Motivation to return to function within the community can be influenced by the previous community role of the patient. A 72-year-old woman who had a CVA had recovered physically to a fairly independent level. She could safely ambulate with a quad cane, and her personal care was independent and safe. She had a resulting aphasia that left her with occasional word-finding difficulties, which increased with fatigue. The occupational therapist noticed an increase of dependence on her family to provide social activities. Her family could not meet this need to the extent the patient seemed to require, so she became irritable with her family and depressed about her lack of social interaction. The occupational therapist suggested she use the senior citizens' services by riding the seniors' bus to the center for a meal, recreation, and social interaction. The patient absolutely refused to consider this possibility. She had previously been the mayor of the city and, during her term of office, had been instrumental in facilitating the development and building of the senior citizen center. She had held a very high-status position in her community and being a very proud person, she was afraid to attend the senior center for fear "someone there might know her." She was also embarrassed by her word-finding problems, although her speech was quite functional. With the patient's unwillingness to attend activities at the senior center, the occupational therapist had to search for other motivational strategies to incorporate into the patient's treatment recommendations.

All the various roles individuals play can be very evident in the home-health setting. Occupational therapists need to face these very important issues as soon as possible in the treatment process in order to understand what motivates us to want to perform certain tasks.

Many times the physical living environment can affect our motivation to participate in health-related activities. One of my job duties includes management of a contract with a local housing authority of a multidisciplinary wellness program. This program is funded by the housing authority, is conducted in several residential apartment buildings, and is free of charge to all the residents who live in the residential building. The program includes a health clinic staffed by a nurse, with a dietician and a social worker providing weekly group education and individual consultation. The occupational therapist provides weekly activity groups, walking groups, and upper extremity exercise groups. As the staff and I have planned together to increase the number of residents participating in the program, we have discovered many variables affecting their behavior. Some elderly residents have expressed fear of the younger disabled residents who live in the facility. Observing differences in generational behavior, the elderly apparently feel afraid and have stated they do not want to leave the security of their apartments, even when it means receiving free, health-related services. Over the last 2 ½ years, we have observed that with the consistent presence of our staff and increasing trust of the residents, the number of people participating in the wellness program has improved. The wellness staff has also learned that providing food is a wonderful motivating factor. In our efforts to provide a total wellness program, we have included proper diet instructions for diabetes, hypertension, and other medically related conditions. One of our most successful techniques has been the dietician and the occupational therapist providing a taste test for various heart-healthy foods. The dietician planned the diet menu consisting of low-fat, low-cholesterol food, and the occupational therapist supervised the residents participating in cooking the heart-healthy menu. The result was an increase of 300 percent participation based on our usual average!

Providing occupational therapy services in the home and community presents numerous challenges. Many times therapists are left feeling like they have to sink or swim. Management's use of motivational strategies with professional staff is as essential as the professional staff's use of motivational strategies with patients. A system of periodic evaluations, joint visits, scheduled meetings, and telephone calls helps convey the message of concern and care for their well-being as professionals. An organized approach to supervision and ongoing management support assists in maintaining wellness for occupational therapists and all health professionals in the multifaceted, fast-changing arena of home and community health.

REFERENCES

American Occupational Therapy Association. The Home and Community Health Task Force. (1994). *Guidelines for occupational therapy practice in home health.* Bethesda, MD: Author.

Steinhauer, M. (1995). *Guidelines for occupational therapy practice in home health.* Bethesda, MD: American Occupational Therapy Association.

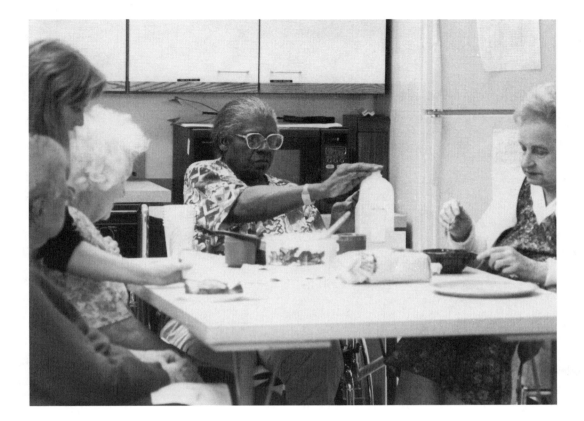

Chapter **8** *Group Programs in a Short-Term Rehabilitation Setting*

Virginia J. Morgan, OTR/L and Paul N. Petrone, MOT/L

Group treatments are used more frequently than ever before in short-term physical disabilities rehabilitation settings. Health care practitioners, responding to changes in reimbursement sources, use group treatment approaches to provide quality therapy at lower costs.

In a short-term rehabilitation hospital, where the average length of stay is 25–30 days, patients participate in a wide variety of individual and group therapy programs. Patients have unique and multiple needs, some of which can best be met on an individual basis and some of which can only be met in a group setting.

Groups are effective in short-term rehabilitation for both clinicians and patients. For the clinician, groups can be time efficient because they can treat more than one patient at a time. Groups can also provide the opportunity to observe and evaluate patients in a setting other than one-on-one treatment. Does a patient attend better in a group setting or have decreased attention? Is the patient more motivated when with peers, more social, less depressed? The

answers to these questions and others can help to effectively direct the course of therapy and determine appropriate discharge plans.

For patients, the benefits are many. Often, patients are concerned about how others perceive them. In a group setting, they can begin making adjustments necessary to accept their new self-image. In a group, patients feel less isolated in their illness and less alone with their problems. A group can provide mutual support and help individuals build confidence and social skills. Groups provide a dynamic whereby patients feel encouraged to do more than they might do alone. They are encouraged to participate more actively in exercise, do more problem solving, and offer options to help others. The group provides an opportunity for nurturing. It often fosters a sense of self-worth, value, and hope. After the group session, patients feel they know each other. The mutual support that began in the group extends outside the group session. The skills learned and the insight gained by participating in group activities prepare patients for their future endeavors and encounters. They have gained the knowledge that they are not alone with their problems, that they can be successful in social situations, and that they can turn to others for support. This better equips patients for situations that arise after discharge, whether they will be in an independent living situation, a supportive environment, or another facility.

CONSIDERATIONS WHEN DEVELOPING A GROUP

Successful groups are those that are carefully planned and developed. Though groups clearly have their utility and benefits, they are not for all patients or all facilities. The development phase determines if a group is indicated. It also determines who will participate in the group; who will run the group; and when, where, and how the group will run.

When developing a group in your facility, it is necessary to consider patients, logistics, and staffing.

- Patients
  - What are the needs of the patient population?
  - Can patients' needs be met in a group setting?
  - Can the patients function successfully in a group setting?

If you determine there are appropriate patients with needs that can be met in a group setting, consider the logistics of running a group.

- Logistics
  - Is there space available to accommodate patients, staff, and equipment for a group?
  - Can the patients' schedules accommodate a new group?
  - What materials will be needed and who will pay for the materials?
  - Is there space to store the materials?

With the need and concrete resources established, consider staffing.

- Staffing
  - Are all appropriate disciplines included in the planning?
  - Are there adequate staff available to run the group?
  - What expectations are there for the group leader(s)?
  - Who will train and supervise the leader(s)?

With all these guidelines addressed, you are well on your way to developing a group. The following is a list of suggestions that we have found helpful in setting up groups in our short-term rehabilitation facility.

- Develop a referral and screening process so patients are appropriately matched to each group and referrals are ongoing.

- Use two leaders, whenever possible, so enough attention can be paid to each group member.

- Try not to rotate leaders more often than once in 3 months. This allows for continuity of the group process. Leaders get to know patients, patients get to know and trust leaders.

- Have patients be part of the decision-making process in groups, when appropriate.

- Be sure groups are fun and interesting so patients will want to come to the session.

- Consider including these techniques: review current events, play physical and mental games, acknowledge patients' birthdays or discharge, use humor.

- Fit the time and place of the group within patient and staff demands of the rehabilitation day.

- Consider ambiance. The environment should be open, airy, friendly, and quiet.

Therapy groups may be led by one or more disciplines and fall into several categories. Types of groups include exercise, functional activities retraining, cognitive/orientation, psychosocial/adjustment, and education.

The following are examples of each type of group.

- Exercise
  - Cardiopulmonary exercise class
  - Stroke upper extremity group
  - Amputee exercise/education group
- Functional retraining
  - Cooking group
  - Functional living skills group
  - Prevocational workshop
- Cognitive/orientation
  - Newsletter group
  - Cognitive/community skills group
  - Current events group
- Psychosocial/adjustment
  - Family stroke discussion group

  - Amputee transition group
  - Oncology support group
- Education
  - Cardiopulmonary energy conservation group
  - Hip education group
  - Wellness group

The following generic group protocol delineates the essential components of a well-planned group:

- Title: Determine appropriately descriptive title.

- Purpose: Define what the group will provide to and accomplish for the patients.

- Objectives: Determine realistic, measurable goals for patients in the group.

- Criteria for referral: Define the capabilities of the patients who will be appropriate to participate in the group.

- Method of referral: Develop a system for staff to refer patients to the group.

- Group size: Determine a minimum and maximum number based on patient needs and abilities, staffing, and space.

- Leadership: Determine how many leaders are required and which disciplines should be involved.

- Leadership training and qualifications: Define expectations of leaders in terms of educational level and group leadership abilities.

- Supervision: Determine who will supervise leaders and frequency of supervision.

- Documentation: Describe method by which information is conveyed from leader to primary therapist; assign responsibility for documenting information in medical record.

- Charges: Follow appropriate fiscal procedures as defined by facility.

- Time and location: State when and where the group will be held.

- Evaluation: Develop a system to determine the effectiveness of the group; determine whether the defined objectives are being met.

- Follow-up: Describe process by which the primary therapist follows up on issues or problems that arise with a patient during a group.

This functional retraining group protocol is based on the previously outlined generic group protocol.

- Title: Functional retraining group

- Purpose:
  - Increase patients' safety awareness and knowledge of energy conservation strategies.
  - Encourage patients to problem solve for their specific needs.
  - Provide opportunity for the sharing of personal experiences and ideas.

- Objectives:
  - Patient will demonstrate good knowledge of safety in the home environment.
  - Patient will demonstrate good knowledge of adaptations to promote energy conservation.
  - Patient will demonstrate problem-solving skills relative to own home environment.

- Criteria for referral:
  - Patient's diagnosis is appropriate for group goals.
  - Patient demonstrates adequate cognitive abilities for group participation.
  - Patient has adequate interaction skills.
  - Patient's behavior would not be disruptive to the group process.
  - Patient has adequate physical endurance for a 1-hour group.
  - Patient is interested in attending the group.

- Method of referral: Primary OTR completes sign-up sheet, files it in group folder, and notifies the group leader.

- Group size: 3–10 members.

- Leadership: Two leaders are required, one from occupational therapy and one from physical therapy.

- Leadership training and qualifications:
  - Leaders are registered or licensed occupational therapists and physical therapists.
  - Leaders demonstrate effective group dynamic skills and communication skills.
  - Leaders demonstrate competency in instruction of safety and energy conservation techniques.

- Supervision: Group leader meets with occupational therapy supervisor during regularly scheduled supervision times to discuss the group process.

◆ Documentation: Leaders note patient's participation and significant observations in group log. Primary therapist is responsible for reading group log and incorporating appropriate information in weekly progress note.

◆ Charges: Leader indicates attendance at group in group log. Primary therapist enters number of group units on charge sheet.

◆ Time and location: Group meets Tuesday and Thursday from 11:00–12:00, 7th floor dining room.

◆ Evaluation: Patients are tested before and after the group on their safety awareness and problem-solving abilities.

◆ Follow-up: Primary therapist communicates with group leader after addressing with patient any issues or problems that arose during group.

In conclusion, group therapy approaches provide appropriate and cost-effective treatment to patients with a wide variety of diagnoses. The use of groups in rehabilitation is a creative approach to meeting the patient's needs while also meeting the demands of the changing health care market.

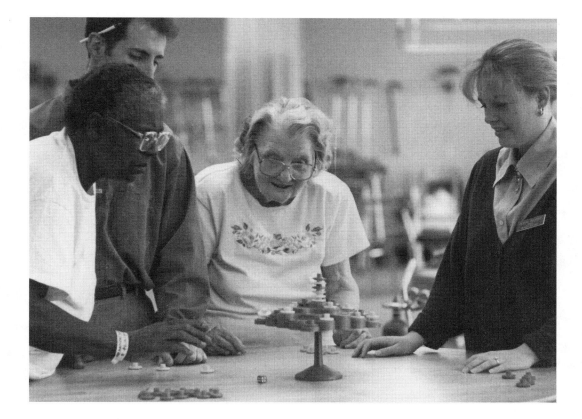

9 *Successful Group Programs in Subacute Rehabilitation*

Karen McCarthy, COTA/L and Martin Proulx, COTA/L

This chapter is based on the knowledge and practical skills we use in the treatment of the geriatric population on a subacute rehabilitation unit. We will share some of the motivational techniques we have found to be successful, as well as describe a few therapeutic groups we feel would work well when incorporated into a subacute treatment milieu.

When discussing a subacute rehabilitation or skilled nursing facility (SNF) unit, it is important to understand the particular population to which we provide treatment. For the purpose of this chapter, the *subacute* or *SNF unit* is described as a facility that furnishes skilled nursing and rehabilitation services on a daily basis. Patients are admitted to this type of facility after staying at least 3 consecutive days on a hospital unit yet requiring longer rehabilitation to increase their independent functional potential beyond their acute stay in the hospital.

The rehabilitation team consists of occupational, physical, and speech therapies, as well as skilled nursing, nutritional, and social services with psychological intervention as needed.

The general population ranges in age from late 60s to mid 90s with long-term goals of increasing independence whether discharged to home, an independent living situation, or a rest/nursing home.

The majority of treatment we provide is in individual sessions, but as skilled therapists we can readily visualize the important impact made by the combination of the individual and group sessions. We can also see the major role groups may play in the overall rehabilitation process.

With backgrounds in psychogeriatric treatment, we commonly use a group setting as a basic treatment modality. Within these groups we are able to achieve targeted goals for the patients involved in occupational therapy.

Unfortunately, the value and outcome of good group treatment appear to be overlooked and underused in the rehabilitation of the geriatric patient in the subacute setting. We are finding it difficult to incorporate skilled group sessions into our daily repertoire of treatments and still remain in compliance with insurance reimbursement guidelines. We hope that this situation will change with the increasing numbers of elderly patients who are covered by HMOs. It is hoped that within the next few years, insurances will acknowledge the value of the group as a viable and cost-effective treatment modality in the subacute setting.

MOTIVATIONAL STRATEGIES

It is important to realize that whether you are treating in an individual or group session, the therapeutic outcomes are strongly influenced by motivational strategies. What is it that motivates a patient to actively participate in treatment and what role does the therapist assume in fostering motivation?

A simple strategy to elicit motivation involves the choice of activities. The treatment content either in a group format or individual session should possess the qualities of a purposeful activity. Selecting an activity that has some significance, value, and interest to the patient may ensure greater involvement in the treatment session. Another motivating factor is to encourage the patient to be involved in designing his or her own treatment. Providing the patient with a thorough understanding of all aspects of his or her targeted goals and treatment may increase his or her potential to achieve them. The more knowledge a patient has regarding his or her current functional status and long-term goals, the better understanding he or she will have of his or her treatment program. The patient will better understand clinical decisions made by the therapists when he or she can see how the decisions relate to personal goals.

We listen to and acknowledge patient concerns and offer support to assist patients in making healthful decisions. Also, remember that each patient is different. Even if their medical cases are similar, your approach should be adapted to meet the cognitive needs of each individual. Simply stated, what works for one patient may not work for another.

Lack of motivation becomes evident when a patient feels that he or she has failed in therapy. It is the therapist's role to assist the patient in identifying realistic goals and to work on techniques to reach those goals. When the patients are able to experience a success in a therapy session, they may be more motivated to continue. We have adopted the rule that we end each session with an activity in which we know the patient will be able to succeed. Therefore the patient ends the session with a positive attitude, which appears to be what patients recall when they discuss their session with nursing staff and family members. Along with building rapport with your patients and their family, it is important to establish a "common ground" in order to facilitate successful treatment.

TALKING THE TALK

We are writing this from our experiences with a geriatric population, and so we are dealing with age-specific examples. The general principles, however, apply equally to any age group. Basically stated, you must be able to speak the same cultural language as your patients in order to truly communicate and therefore, motivate.

Yearly, our schools produce classes of occupational therapists for whom even the Vietnam conflict is often vague, ancient history. For the current geriatric population, mainly born in the first 2 decades of the 20th century, certain events, names, dates, and cultural trends form an overwhelmingly powerful and relevant background of shared experiences. The Great Depression, the World Wars, the presidency of Franklin Roosevelt, the New Deal, rationing—all these things form a lexicon of meaning and common memory for the patients we treat. A geriatric patient who is isolated at home or who is institutionalized is often surrounded by young caregivers who know almost nothing of the time or the historical era from which their charges have sprung. In order to encourage our patients to "walk the walk"—participate in their therapy—we need to learn their cultural language and "talk the talk."

A NEW WAR TO FIGHT

Alex was admitted to this facility suffering from an exacerbation of his chronic pulmonary disease. He had no family in the area, his wife had died years ago, they had no children, and his siblings lived in another state. Alex was described as "an isolated, anxious, needy man."

The day of his admission, Alex sat on his bedside in a four-bed dorm, staring out into the noisy corridor with large, frightened-looking eyes. No doubt he heard lots of rap and rock music from nearby radios and televisions. No doubt he heard bits of conversation from nearby staff full of words he did not understand, the workday lingo of the nursing home, medical terminology, references to "O.J." or "Internet"—all of these things floated past him; the air smelled of disinfectant and resounded with the clash of trays being returned to the breakfast cart.

Alex initially refused to wash or dress, only wanting to "get the hell out of here." He wanted to see the "boss of the kitchen" to complain about his breakfast. An anxious man indeed.

His chart mentioned a history of malaria. As is typical, there was no elaboration of this. Neither was there a social history to relate how this man had spent his life, what frightened him, what had importance to him. There was a date of birth listed. Anyone with a working knowledge of 20th-century American history could place his life against a time line of events. Anyone wishing to get to know Alex, wishing to find out what might motivate him, would need to be able to sit and talk with him in terms he would understand.

"Alex, you had malaria? How did you get that?"

"I caught it in North Africa, during the war." Instantly the picture begins to form of this man and his life experience. Some basic knowledge and the right series of questions can now begin to flesh out the picture, and there is a crack in the dam.

Our therapy sessions fell into a pattern. I approached him initially as a helper, to empty his urinal, or to inquire if he felt warm enough. After innocuous remarks about weather, one of us—it did not seem to matter who—began with war reminiscences. I allowed him to steer the conversation, in case there were memories he wished to avoid. To him, I repeatedly made it clear that I was impressed, that I was proud, that I was grateful for his service to our country. He had fought across Africa and then into Sicily and up the Italian peninsula. He gave dates, places, battles, and leaders in detail, although he could not locate his socks this morning and was vague about what he had for supper last night.

Alex made it clear, as well, that he was impressed and pleased that such a young man could seem so interested and knowledgeable regarding events of 50 years past. After we chatted for a bit, he was willing to walk to the rehabilitation room, despite chronic shortness of breath. He participated consistently in exercises that were obviously difficult for him. Did I detect in his eyes a glint of determined pride?—the same pride that had impelled him as a young man to sacrifice his health fighting Nazis? These are subjective questions, but results say much.

Alex still wants to get "the hell out of here" and will probably make it to a rest home. His participation in therapy is enabling him to gain sufficient strength and self-confidence to leave this skilled nursing facility and go to a smaller, quieter, homelike setting. Those clinical-sounding goals—"maximize functional capabilities" and "discharge to a less restrictive setting"—may indeed be achieved. Other, subtler things also appear to be happening during the therapy sessions. "Quality of life," renewed purpose, and the sense of past accomplishments and future possibilities—if these can be imparted in some degree to our patients—serve as vital adjuncts to things like increased muscle strength and improved balance.

USE OF GROUP TREATMENT

If the individual treatment session outcomes can be so strongly influenced by simple motivational strategies, it only makes sense that the skilled group session may have an even more profound influence. A well-designed and implemented group can decrease the patients' sense of loneliness, isolation, and fearfulness around the aspects of their rehabilitation. Interacting with others facing similar life issues provides mutual reinforcement and encouragement for active participation in treatments that are frequently difficult and painful.

The value of group treatment should not be overlooked by occupational therapists who work in the subacute rehabilitation setting. The group setting provides a forum in which patients can practice the skills they are striving to acquire or those they have attained in the individual session. The group also allows its members to relate to other patients who not only share a common cultural heritage and life span, but also share common concerns and similar goals. The group becomes a source of support and peer feedback significant to the rehabilitation process. The patients are able to develop relationships within the group structure that may not occur in individual sessions. As a result, patients often become productive members of the unit community. Friendship and support often continue after the session has been completed. We have found that these factors increase the patients' motivation to actively participate in therapy, thus expediting the rehabilitation process and possibly shortening the length of time necessary for recuperation, which should be of value to the insurance companies paying for treatment. When patients become motivated to help others and to assume an active role in their treatment, they also increase their self-esteem and sense of self-worth by regaining control over important aspects of their daily lives.

INCORPORATING GROUP TREATMENT

Once a therapist decides to include the group session as a basic modality in the subacute treatment milieu, it becomes important to do some research in order to decide which groups will be the most beneficial to the current rehabilitation schedule. A well-designed group is essential to meeting the specific goals of each member, as well as to remaining in compliance with professional ethics and with company treatment values and policies.

Before using a group format, a protocol should be in place to ensure that all leaders are using the same basic concepts to help the group strive to achieve designated goals. Although the therapists' general leadership styles may vary, the group outcomes should be consistent. It is important to develop group protocols prior to using group treatment to assist the therapist in designing and implementing therapeutic groups to

meet the needs of patients involved in treatment and to facilitate documentation and demonstration of the effectiveness of group treatment to administrators, rehabilitation coordinators, and insurance companies.

The group protocol is a detailed outline of a therapeutic group planned for a targeted patient population. When selecting what treatment aspects will be addressed by the group, the therapist must decide what performance areas or performance components the patient needs to improve. Some patients may have more than one area that is deficient. It is here that a well-prepared, skilled group leader is able to select purposeful activities that address several of these areas or components at one time.

Although each section of the protocol is important to address, we have included only a few basic points to consider.

- The *purpose of the group* describes the intent of the group and should include the group's long-term goals and the activities used to achieve them.

- The *group membership criteria* should be as detailed as possible. Diagnostic factors, functional levels, and appropriate characteristics of group members are included in this section.

- The *group rationale and goals* are covered in the next section. The short-term goals of the group session are addressed and should be stated in measurable terms. Goals that are well-written will assist the therapist in planning each session and will simplify documentation of patient progress. This area should also explain your reasons for choosing specific goals. These goals should relate to the targeted goals of the group members.

GETTING STARTED

To avoid frustration and failure, start with the simplest groups. Using your protocol, take inventory of the clinic and staff resources and start from there. Make sure you are well-prepared before attempting group treatment. The two easiest groups to initiate are the upper extremity strengthening and the meal preparation/cooking groups.

Most clinics have the basic equipment: Theraband, balloons, balls, canes, and weights that can be used in a great exercise/strengthening group. Add some music (from the patients' era, of course) and the creative energy of the therapist, and you can have a very successful, well-attended group.

The meal preparation/cooking group can also be set up fairly inexpensively. With the use of a burner or toaster oven, a few kitchen implements, and a kitchen cart, you can create a simple but therapeutic group. As the administrator sees the success and viability of such a treatment modality, as well as the billable units that can be generated, you may be able to procure a kitchen area for your group as well as other therapeutic interventions.

Another approach you may want to research is that of the educational group model. We found a cardiac rehabilitation group based on this model in three facilities we surveyed. All three are having great success with these groups after a great deal of preparation prior to the group's implementation. The main objectives are to educate patients and families about cardiac function and dysfunction. The areas of energy conservation, stress management, and relaxation techniques are also addressed using a variety of interventions.

The stroke group is also based on the educational approach. This group combines discussion and support around the dysfunction as well as functional techniques for the patient and family members.

These last two groups mentioned were led by interdisciplinary coleaders. A combination of staff from OT, PT, and nursing assists in providing more consistent follow-up with the patients after the group has dispersed. It also allows for a more well-rounded group session, where the patients have access to more than one discipline to assist in making better decisions pertaining to their rehabilitation.

THE POWER OF GROUP TREATMENT

Mary is a 70-year-old, divorced female admitted to this facility with a multitude of diagnoses, including decreased activity tolerance, congestive heart failure, pneumonia, chronic obstructive pulmonary disease, and morbid obesity. Information from the medical chart was sparse, containing no other family or social history, and very little documented progress of previous rehabilitation. The chart did state, however, that the "pt. appears depressed" and "unmotivated at times." Mary was admitted to a three-bed dorm with one other roommate.

Mary arrived at the facility after spending 10 days on an acute unit. Her doctor ordered occupational, physical, and speech therapy evaluations with a long-term goal of returning home. Rehabilitation potential upon discharge from the hospital seemed poor, but she wanted to return home, and, therefore, a goal of going home was established. Mary was evaluated and placed on an active program. She was unable to go supine or sit without maximum assistance of two. She was dependent on two staff persons to transfer from bed to chair. Mary's short-term goal was to wash her face and hands at the edge of her bed. We had a long way to go. During the evaluation process, it was determined that Mary would require intensive intervention to meet the long-term goal of discharge home. The first treatment session was shorter than I anticipated, secondary to her decreased endurance and apparent lack of motivation. I tried all the therapeutic "tricks," but I couldn't get Mary to participate.

During the next week, I noticed that if I just spent time talking with Mary (especially about cats) before we attempted to perform the assigned task, she appeared to be more at ease and readily accepted her therapy. Mary required short treatment sessions dispersed throughout the day due to her medical condition, poor endurance, and the fact that she fatigued quickly.

With carefully selected questions, I was able to develop a social history and, at the same time, rapport with Mary. She told me that she was 1 of 11 siblings, had an eighth-grade education, and dropped out of school to help support the family. Mary was married but that ended in divorce and she had no children. Prior to her hospitalization, she lived in a housing complex for the elderly with services from the Visiting Nurses Association. Her sister lived across the hall, but there was no social contact between the two. Mary had few leisure interests, spending most of the day watching the television, and rarely left her apartment.

As therapy slowly progressed, Mary often stated "This is too hard to do; why should I, I'm not going anywhere, I don't care." She needed much encouragement to wash her face and hands. It was apparent that she had very low self-esteem, which also interfered with our treatment sessions. Mary required constant encouragement to become involved in even the simplest of tasks. I attempted to have Mary choose her own treatments, but even that was too difficult at this time. I encouraged Mary to choose activities that we could incorporate into our sessions, but this attempt also failed.

The plan remained that of discharge home, living alone with services as needed, but it appeared that Mary was unsure of this. She would often give excuses for her inability to complete tasks needed for discharge. I was beginning to feel that she was sabotaging her discharge despite her stated desire to the contrary.

One day Mary got a new roommate and assumed the role of "welcome wagon." When I entered her room for our daily therapy session, I saw Mary as I have never seen her before. She had a purpose. Mary introduced me to her new friend. I explained my role to this new patient and invited Mary to explain what we did in therapy. She not only described what we did in therapy, but she also invited her roommate (Ann) to join us in exercising.

It was amazing to witness Mary in her new role. Although Mary was making steady but slow progress, she had a new spark. She was needed by someone. The majority of Mary's therapy sessions continued to take place in her room, including ADL, functional transfers, and the upper body exercise program. Mary did not want to leave the security of her room or the oxygen machine (which she was on continually), despite my reassurances that the portable oxygen would be sufficient and a change of scenery would do her a world of good.

Mary's roommate was now mobile, venturing out of their room, attending the upper body exercise group three times weekly. With much encouragement from me and other staff and the insistence of Ann, Mary attended her first off-unit group. Much to her surprise, she liked it. Not long after that first group, Mary participated in leading her favorite exercise. She received a rousing round of applause and positive feedback from her peers. If the group leaders forgot to do her exercise, she would speak up and remind us. She assumed the role of encouraging the other patients to attend the groups. She would actually leave her room and wheel around, gathering group members. Her active participation in daily therapy was also improving, her endurance was actually increasing, and

she would ask to go to the clinic or the rehabilitation kitchen to make lunch with the others. Was it my imagination—were these group interactions actually assisting Mary in her rehabilitation?

As her physical health improved, she was weaned off her oxygen dependency. She progressed in her ADL skills, actually caring about what she looked like and what she wore when she went to her groups. She had progressed to minimal assistance in her transfers with a walker, minimal assistance in the bathroom for her ADL, and she was ambulating with a walker and minimal assistance with her rehabilitation technicians. She was also independent in wheelchair mobility. Her discharge plans had changed. She decided with her social worker that living independently was not an option for her due to her medical condition. She really did not want to leave the nursing home. Mary appeared to be somewhat relieved with this decision and was transferred off the rehabilitation unit to the extended unit at the facility.

Mary is rooming with two other very active residents in the nursing home and is rarely found in her room. She is one of the most social residents. She can be found attending all of the scheduled groups and socializing when there is no group. She also encourages other patients to do the same. Mary has developed a great sense of humor and a sense of pride in her ability to help other residents.

Of course I have no scientific proof that the power of group treatment motivated this once very sick, lonely lady to actively participate in her rehabilitation. All I have is her word and her belief that the groups keep her healthy and happy.

SUMMARY

As group leaders, we have observed group members motivating one another as the cohesiveness of the group progresses. This interaction alleviates some of the therapists' burden to motivate the patients for treatment. While working with the psychiatric population, it was common for us to use various examples and personal life experiences to encourage patient participation. This is one strategy that we do not readily observe in the field of physical dysfunction. As skilled therapists, we should be prepared to treat patients holistically, including whatever motivational factors it takes to achieve the patients' greatest potential.

We have attempted, in this chapter, to express our views on the importance of group treatment. We acknowledge that in realistic, practical terms, our therapy modalities need to be acceptable for billing and reimbursement. But we also know that incorporating individual and group treatment sessions increases the patients' potential and motivation to actively participate in their treatment. The group concepts we have suggested are specifically designed to address patients' individual, billable goals. The group formats we have discussed reinforce motivation to achieve these goals. It is important for occupational therapists to use every tool at their disposal in order to maximize the chances of successful treatment outcomes. We hope that insurance providers for subacute rehabilitation services will begin to

recognize the validity of the group treatment approach and realize that group treatment may ultimately prove to be among the most cost-effective measures we can provide.

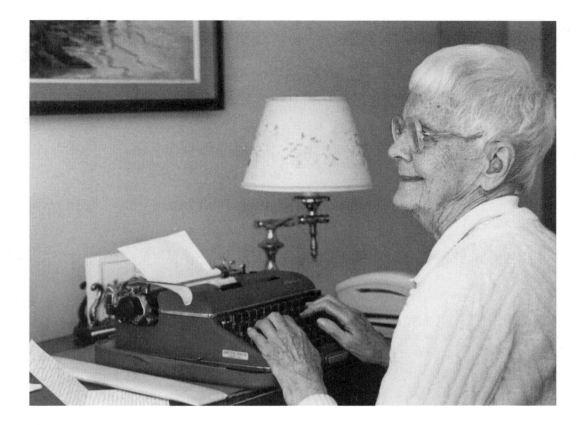

10 Impact of Financial Status, Values, and Attitudes on Motivation for Rehabilitation

Paul J. Goldberg, MSW, LICSW and Rick Fentin, MEd, CFP

INTRODUCTION

Feelings about money and personal financial status are arguably two of the most emotionally charged issues in our culture. Although most people are reluctant to talk about their finances, we often partially measure our self-worth by the amount of money we make, the size of our house, the kind of car we drive, or how much savings we have in the bank. These measurements and evaluations are based not only on what we actually have but also, more importantly, on how we perceive what we have with respect to our own wealth or poverty. Money and our feelings about financial status powerfully affect our options and the choices we make in life.

While we can point to no research directly linking motivation for rehabilitation with financial issues, our experience suggests that personal financial status as well as attitudes toward money have an important influence on a client's acceptance of and involvement with health care services. The benefits and eligibility requirements of public and private insurances and other social service programs may influence a client's decisions regarding rehabilitation. The following discussion is intended to raise therapists' awareness of what we call the "informal" financial issues affecting the rehabilitation of senior citizens (attitudes, perceptions, and personal meaning of financial resources) and the "formal" influences (availability of and access to financial resources, insurance programs, and social services). There is a great deal of overlap between these two spheres. Decisions about rehabilitation are forged by individual and family financial values, beliefs, and attitudes as well as by the financial parameters of care defined by our health care institutions.

FORMAL ISSUES: FINANCIAL RESOURCES

There are three major types of resources that compose an individual's endowment to access health care: (1) individual/family income and assets, (2) health-related social services for which the individual is eligible, and (3) health insurances.

Through local councils on aging and federal aging programs, many communities offer elders social services and some health care. These programs include health screenings (e.g., vision, hearing, diabetes), health education groups, adult day health programs, and transportation to medical appointments. Of these services, transportation (discussed below) has the most bearing on access to rehabilitation.

Federal, state, and private insurance programs for geriatric clients are undergoing almost constant review and change. Services, eligibility rules, prices, and funding levels are being revised to cope with the growing need and increased cost of elder health care. For clients whose health insurance and supplementary plans pay for 100 percent of their care, or for individuals who are sufficiently affluent, the cost of rehabilitation services may not be of concern. But for individuals incurring insurance copayments or whose insurance covers little or no rehabilitation, the out-of-pocket financial impact may be very significant.

How large a copayment, if any, a client will be required to pay is determined by the type of insurance and the setting (inpatient hospital, home care, outpatient, or skilled nursing facility) in which services are delivered. As discussion of all insurance programs and social services available to seniors is not possible, we have selected Medicare, Medicaid, and the expanding managed care model of insurance for review.

MEDICARE

Medicare is a federal health insurance program for individuals who have contributed to Social Security or railroad retirement funds or are eligible because of Medicare-qualified government employment. Although disabled individuals and others under age 65 may receive these benefits, the vast majority of beneficiaries are over age 65. Because Medicare is based on financial contributions made while gainfully employed, it is not a needs-based program and has no financial eligibility requirements.

Hospital Setting

In an acute or rehabilitation hospital, patients must pay a $736 deductible before Medicare payments are applied. (This deductible is for 1996. It changes annually based on cost-of-living calculations. All figures quoted are for 1996 only.) There is a substantial copayment after 60 days of hospitalization ($184/day) and an increased copayment ($368/day) after 90 days of hospital care. (An individual has 60 lifetime reserve days for which Medicare pays all but $368/day. Once these days are used up, the benefit ends.) With today's high costs of hospitalization, the deductible is usually incurred on admission day. In general, a client's motivation to regain health and a baseline level of functioning appears to outweigh any financial considerations regarding participation in rehabilitation services. Since there is such a high acuity level necessary for hospital admission and lengths of stay are so brief, patients typically are more focused on recovery than on financial concerns.

Home-Health Setting

In a home-health setting, such as a visiting nurse agency, Medicare currently pays for 100 percent of the skilled rehabilitation services. Generally, financial considerations do not affect a client's decisions regarding care. However, there is a 20 percent copayment for such durable medical equipment as wheelchairs and walkers, and no insurance coverage for weights, sliding boards, sock reachers, and bathroom equipment (tub chairs, grab bars, and raised toilet seats). For those clients whose income or assets are sufficiently small, the copayment or out-of-pocket expense for this equipment or related household adaptations may be prohibitive. Often, home-care clients will directly state that the cost of the equipment is beyond their means. The inability to afford such low-cost items as a basket attached to a walker, for example, can become a significant safety concern. In the kitchen, without the basket to transport items to the table, a client may forego using his or her walker in order to transport items in his or her hands, thus risking a serious fall.

Outpatient Hospital Setting

Medicare requires a 20 percent copayment for all rehabilitation services. Durable medical equipment follows the financial guidelines outlined in the home-health section. One of the most revealing clinical situations in terms of observing the financial impact on services occurs when a client is being prepared to "graduate" from in-home rehabilitation to outpatient care. Therapists report that when some clients are told they will have to pay for services, their faces drop. They will couch their opposition to the copayment by saying, "It's too difficult to get to the clinic," or "I have nobody to take me." Others will say they are too tired to leave their home, or that it is too much of a difficulty to go to an outpatient appointment. An experienced therapist who knows the client well will be able to discern the legitimacy of these excuses.

Many clients are referred to outpatient rehabilitation without being aware of the copayment. Between the second and fourth clinic visit they may ask, "Is this being covered by Medicare?" Soon after, they may begin skipping clinic visits or may call the clinic to say, "I'm feeling a lot better now and don't think I need any more therapy." This can be very frustrating for the therapist.

Another factor that clearly affects a client's use of outpatient rehabilitation is the availability of transportation. Medicare does not pay for transportation to and from medical appointments. Out-of-pocket expenses for a client may include not only the transportation itself, but also the cost of an escort, if needed. Many communities provide transportation and escort services for a nominal fee or for free. If these services are not easily accessible (e.g., a chair van making many stops before a frail client is delivered to the outpatient facility) or not available at all, access to rehabilitation services will be thwarted.

Skilled Nursing Facility

In a skilled nursing home setting, Medicare and medigap plans pay none of the long-term nursing home costs.

These costs can average between $30,000 and $70,000 per year. For clients who are discharged from a hospital and go to a skilled nursing facility, Medicare will pay for 20 days of care before the client begins to incur a $92/day copayment. After 100 days, Medicare and medigap plans pays nothing for a skilled nursing facility.

For clients and families who face long-term care in a skilled nursing facility, financial considerations appear to have more of a bearing on how long a client or family tries to defer admission than on whether or not to accept rehabilitation services once admitted. Deferring admission is frequently influenced by how much financial planning the client/family did to legally protect their assets from being depleted. Financial considerations, however, may affect clients entering a skilled nursing facility from a hospital and expecting to return home. A 78-year-old woman had been caring for her 96-year-old husband, who had repeatedly fallen over a 2-year period, fracturing his leg or pelvis on three separate occasions. Each time he fell, he was admitted to an acute facility, and on the occasions when he sustained a fracture, he was then transferred to a rehabilitation hospital and finally to a nursing home. After his last nursing home admission, his wife insisted that he return home before the full Medicare benefits expired. The husband was in total agreement with this plan, even though he had not completed his course of rehabilitation at the time of discharge. Efforts on the part of the staff to convince him to stay were ignored by both client and spouse and

reflected their attitude toward their financial status (discussed below).

MEDICAID

The Program

The federal/state Medicaid program is available to individuals over age 65 with very limited income and assets (currently $614/month income and $2,000 assets for an individual). Clients whose income exceeds the eligibility level may still qualify for Medicaid if they "spend down" their income and assets by subtracting any out-of-pocket medically related expenses from their current income or assets.

Hospital, Home-Health, and Outpatient Settings

Medicaid pays for 100 percent of rehabilitation services in these settings. Coverage for durable medical equipment varies from state to state. In Massachusetts, Medicaid will currently pay for ambulatory devices, sliding boards, tub seats, grab bars, and raised toilet seats. If individuals on Medicaid are indigent, denial of benefits for durable medical equipment is a barrier for continued rehabilitation. The client must then rely on donated equipment obtained informally or through social service agencies.

Skilled Nursing Facility

Medicaid will pay 100 percent of long-term-care expenditures in a nursing home. (Aside from this program, only personal assets and private long-term-care insurance are available for nursing home costs.) Once a client is admitted to a nursing home, if Medicaid is the primary insurance, there is no financial impact on services offered.

INSTITUTIONAL CONSTRAINTS ON SERVICES AND MANAGED CARE

Health care providers have a strong influence on the delivery of rehabilitation services. Health care institutions must follow insurance guidelines regarding the appropriateness of services to be provided. In an ideal world, a client's need for services and not his or her insurance plan would determine the level of services provided. Health care organizations, however, must heed the laws of economics and fiscal responsibility, and have long lived with utilization review committees that determine whether or not insurance criteria for continued payment for services are being met. Particularly in today's highly competitive health care environment, financial considerations figure prominently in decision making regarding the frequency and duration of services provided.

Clients with managed care insurance also have case managers involved in the decision-making process, adding yet another dimension of fiscal accountability. Managed Medicare insurance is a rapidly growing option among Medicare recipients, who are drawn to join these programs because they eliminate all traditional Medicare copayments. Insurance companies are paid a fixed sum of money per client from Medicare

(the Health Care Finance Administration) with the expectation they can provide comprehensive care for less than this fixed sum and thus show a financial gain. If health costs exceed the amount allocated, they lose money on the client.

Ideally, this arrangement builds in incentives for providers to offer clients more education and preventive care to keep them as healthy as possible and out of expensive emergency departments and acute care facilities. The verdict is still out as to whether these managed Medicare programs save money and maintain the same quality of health care that clients enjoyed with their traditional Medicare benefits. HMOs have claimed quality and health care outcomes are not compromised as costs of care are reduced. Anecdotal information suggests that costs are at times reduced by making access to services more difficult, with case managers denying services that the client, and, sometimes, the therapist feel are needed.

There also have been some disturbing reports that a few managed care organizations have required providers (doctors and psychologists) to sign contractual agreements forbidding them from informing a client of recommended continued treatment if the case manager determined that no further treatment was necessary or justified. Providers also were forbidden to reveal the existence of this contractual arrangement to their clients. Some clinicians claim to have been "blackballed" from preferred provider lists because they advocated for continued or increased services on their client's behalf. Providers have organized legal challenges to these practices. In Massachusetts, legislation has recently passed banning such contractual arrangements.

The dilemma rehabilitation therapists potentially face in dealing with managed care entities is how to reconcile one's role as an independent professional with today's funding realities, which focus on the bottom line. Therapists are faced with ethical concerns about a client's right to knowledge regarding his or her treatment and the potential health effects on the client of discontinuation of care.

As the health care field moves toward a managed care model, the issue of financial cost versus potential benefit from rehabilitation will become more prominent. Decisions about whether rehabilitation services should be provided, and if so, what will be their frequency and duration, will increasingly be made in partnership among the case manager, client, and therapist.

For elderly clients and families whose lives are distressed and disrupted by illness and the adjustments in lifestyle that caregiving entails, there may be little energy left to advocate with insurance companies for needed rehabilitation services if these services have been denied. As one caregiver daughter said regarding her efforts to obtain additional services for her mother with whom she lived, "I have to fight for everything that I get." This can become so exhausting that many families eventually give up.

INFORMAL ISSUES: PERSONAL VALUES, PERCEPTIONS, AND ATTITUDES ABOUT MONEY AND FINANCES

Clients' and families' personal values, perceptions, and attitudes about money may play a significant role in a successful rehabilitation program. An objective analysis of financial resources is important, but many times financial decisions are made based on a client's perception of his or her situation as judged by a personal internal standard and influenced by deep-seated fears and desires.

When an elderly client enters a nursing home, the client's family is frequently quite fearful of depleting all the assets. A healthy spouse may worry about having little to live on, particularly if the client is suffering from a long-standing, chronic illness and the spouse has witnessed a steady outflow of medical expenses. These concerns may lead to unsound health care decisions, as in the case of the 96-year-old man who left the nursing home against medical advice. What motivated him and his wife to make this decision for early discharge? One factor appears to be that rehabilitation services were bundled with the total expense of nursing home care, and it did not seem worth their while to accept the whole package of care. They also appeared to have a limited understanding and appreciation of rehabilitation services, undervaluing the benefit of continued therapy and not feeling the additional gains in safety were worth the additional copayment expense. There was an attitude of fatalism and acceptance of the condition. The value of money to this couple and others of their generation has been tempered by living through the Depression. Money was crucial for survival and was not spent on "frivolities."

Clients not born in the United States may have a very different understanding of social welfare programs such as Social Security and Medicare. Lack of information or misinformation about social welfare benefits may create a cultural barrier to using these entitlements. One elderly African American man, seen at home, had worked most of his adult life as an auto mechanic. He was born and raised in Barbados and had never applied to receive Social Security or Medicare. He had no use for "government handouts." After several discussions, he understood that Social Security and Medicare were earned benefits that he was entitled to because of his many years of employment. Finally, he reluctantly allowed the application process for Social Security and Medicare to go forward and he was able to receive more comprehensive services. As we increasingly become a society of cultural diversity, we will need to attend more to similar issues.

The hesitancy for many individuals and families to take what they perceive as government "charity" or "welfare" applies particularly to accessing Medicaid benefits. Some families are extremely proud and feel it is the obligation of a "good family" to take care of their own. Other clients choose not to apply for benefits because they do not want to go through what they consider a demeaning application process during which they must reveal their financial status and provide other personal information.

THE RAINY DAY SYNDROME

The client's or spouse's ability to weigh the relative benefits of therapy versus its financial costs is sometimes impaired by cognitive deficits either may exhibit. Two sisters, aged 97 and 89, living together and having considerable inherited wealth, continue to see themselves as poor because they have no recollection of having received their inheritance nor appreciation of its present worth. They held onto their perceived limited assets and income for a "rainy day."

Even the most cognitively intact elders, those well into their 80s or 90s, may be loathe to spend money on services in order to preserve funds for a "rainy day." Financial resources are charged with strong emotions. It is difficult and painful for them to reconcile themselves to coming to life's end. By not acknowledging that the "rainy day" has arrived, they can hold onto the illusion they still have a long future. More significantly, holding onto these funds allows piece of mind in the waning years of an elder's life, as it symbolizes the ability to provide for an emergency contingency. Furthermore, many elderly parents express strong desires to leave an inheritance for their children and to never, never be financially dependent upon them. Dwindling resources threaten their autonomy and self-esteem.

Financial planners note the significant difference in mind-set regarding money matters between senior citizens and their children. Contrasted with the "accumulation mode" of the younger generation is the "spend-down mode" of older clients who have a fixed-income mentality, realizing that they can no longer change jobs or put in additional work hours to replace depleting assets. A grave fear expressed by many senior citizens is that of living too long and running out of money.

Adult children have their own financial issues to weigh. The "Sandwich Generation," struggling to attend simultaneously to ailing parents and dependent children, must confront the dilemma of financially supporting their parents and encouraging them to spend their own resources on health care, or discouraging outlays of money to preserve their personal wealth and family inheritance. Adult children often suffer the "triage effect" of having to decide whether to put a new wing on the house, send Johnny to college, or put mom in a nursing home. The pressures, guilt, and anxiety can be overwhelming.

The financial pressures on senior citizens, their families, and the programs that provide elderly services are constantly increasing. The over-85 age group, the fastest-growing segment of the U.S. population, also has the highest percentage of people living below the poverty line. Most nursing home residents deplete their entire life savings and that of their spouse before the end of their first year in residence. Many times clients go into nursing homes "too soon" due to lack of financial and family support in the community, or, conversely, elderly parents and spouses are kept at home "too long" before placement in a nursing home because children or spouses want to preserve assets and inheritances through wealth transfer techniques. One very caring and attentive man looking out for his ailing mother, who had suffered a

stroke 15 years before and had become increasingly debilitated, dragged his feet for a year before placing her in a nursing home. Though he knew she needed institutional care and was unsafe at home, she had some assets, and he knew it would all be used up on her nursing home care.

QUESTIONS TO CONSIDER

Clinicians exploring the issue of finances with geriatric clients and families may encounter strong and seemingly unpredictable reactions, because money concerns are rarely openly discussed. Geriatric care managers in meetings with seniors citizens and their families recognize that financial concerns are disguised beneath many of their clients' questions, comments, and decisions. Professionals working with geriatric clients might find it useful to discuss these questions with them, their families, and social service staff at the beginning of a treatment program in order to make the financial dynamics more explicit.

- Do you have insurance? What is your understanding of what the insurance will cover and what expenses you will have?
- Do you know what you are entitled to?
- Will it be a financial hardship to you or your family for you to participate in therapy?
- What value do you feel the therapy has? Do you think it is worth the cost?
- Do you have other plans for the money?

SUMMARY

The way financial considerations affect motivation for rehabilitation can be straightforward or extremely subtle. We define motivation in a broad way, pertaining not just to the client but also to institutional barriers impeding access to services and financial incentives influencing service providers. Relevant factors include a client's income, assets, type of health insurance, and setting in which services are delivered as well as the client's and family's values, attitudes, and perceptions about money. Rehabilitation professionals who are puzzled by the lack of rehabilitation use or progress by clients should not ignore financial issues as a possible explanation for problems. A referral or consultation with social services may be of benefit when one suspects that financial considerations are affecting a client's use of rehabilitation services. Although beliefs and attitudes toward money may not always be amenable to change, an appreciation of how the factors discussed above affect a client's and family's decision-making process can diminish frustration among professional caregivers and increase one's respect for and understanding of the many factors involved in a successful rehabilitation program.

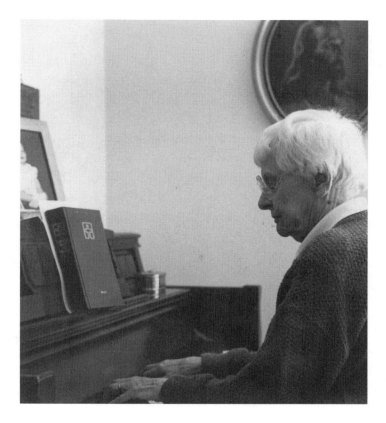

11 *Faith and Religion in Geriatric Rehabilitation*

John D. Weagraff, Jr., PsyD, PhD

*Wholly unprepared, we embark upon the second half of life. ...
Worse still, we take this step with the false assumption that
our truths and ideals will serve us as hitherto. But we cannot live
the afternoon of life according to the programme of life's morning:
for what in the morning of life was true will at evening have
become a lie.*

—Carl Gustave Jung

RELIGION, REHABILITATION, AND THE QUESTION OF MEANING

The relevance of a person's faith and religion as a motivational factor in the rehabilitation process is coming into view for rehabilitation specialists. This occurs as the field articulates and embraces a holistic perspective that attends to the physical, psychological, social, and spiritual dimensions of personhood as fundamental to one's work.

Almost 40 years ago Bateson (1956) pointed out that an occupational therapist's ability to affect change in a person's life was largely contingent on his or her ability to negotiate the manner in which the rehabilitative activity was incorporated within the meaningful intentionality of the person. Since that time there has been a gradual amplification of Bateson's initial insight (Englehardt, 1977) into a relatively clear vision that beliefs and values bear directly on people's ability to engage in and use the interventions offered to them. Most recently, Helfrich and Kielhofner (1994) have begun to speak

the language of "volitional narratives." They note that persons "organize their self-knowledge and choices through narratives, that is, the stories they tell themselves and others" (p. 320). Rosenfeld (1993), in a similar vein, emphasizes the need to integrate function, purpose, and life context in the rehabilitative process, which brings into focus the subjective intentionality of the person as critical to his or her movement through a situational or life crisis.

These developments within the field of occupational therapy parallel significant developments in the understanding of the religious life of persons over the past couple of decades. Under the general rubric of "faith development theory," a number of researchers and practitioners (Fowler, 1981; Fowler, Nipkow, & Schweitzer, 1991; Kegan, 1980; McDargh, 1983) have taken the constructive developmental theories of Piaget and Kohlberg into the realm of faith. They have effected what might be termed a "turn to the subject" such that attention is focused on faith as a "verb" rather than a "noun." In this perspective, the meaning and significance of faith is understood in reference to emergent psychological processes (cognitive, emotional, moral, and spiritual) through which the person constructs and reconstructs his or her world. Faith, then, is intrinsically a dynamic process. It is manifest in increasingly differentiated accounts of self and self in relation to others over the course of the life span. The focus is much less on understanding the substance of doctrine or creed objectively and much more on understanding how and in what manner the person's capacity for religious meaning-making enables him or her to organize his or her experience. The adequacy of a person's faith is measured less in reference to religious authority and more in reference to the manner in which it mediates a constructive response to the challenges of life.

This "constructive" shift provides a conceptual framework within which to articulate the specific manner in which faith may figure as a motivational factor in rehabilitation. Meaning-making is constitutive of human engagement with personal and interpersonal experiences. Whether challenged by the task of negotiating various life transitions or coping with the crises of illness and injury, the human response is to enter into that experience by making sense of it according to individual resources and capacities.

The language of faith and religion simply represents a medium through which some persons construct and articulate their "volitional narratives." For these persons, the relative success with which they meet various life crises and use the resources made available to them may depend on their capacity to

come to terms with the experience in terms of the values, beliefs, and rites of their religious tradition.

AGING, ILLNESS, AND THE CRISIS OF MEANING

Kegan (1983, 1994) has noted that meaning-making is not simply a matter of active engagement but it is also *developmental* in character. The press of life is such that the constructions of value and belief that mediated a sense of identity and relationship at one time may be found wanting with the presentation of new challenges and crises. A crisis of meaning occurs as persons find themselves confronted with the challenge of making sense of new experiences, particularly those that represent fundamental challenges to previous identity formations.

A substantial literature exists that establishes that the transition to elder status, the process of aging itself, and the experience of illness and injury constitute fundamental challenges to personal identity and meaning. The specter of death and the reality of losses, personal and social, invite a contest between "ego-integrity" and "despair" (Erikson, 1950). These themes express the basic tension of aging as a life stage. The maintenance of a sense of integrity and identity when confronted with these challenges to one's sense of mastery and competence may well depend upon becoming a master of one's own meaning.

Heinz (1994) has noted that the fundamental task of old age is, at its core, a spiritual one whether this is expressed in overtly religious language or not. While men and women may gradually have to let go of previous identities organized around the tasks associated with work and raising a family, they have yet to do the "work of culture." This work unfolds as the press of existence in the second half of life invites them to actively engage in the process of recollecting and finishing the story of their lives. This process of "finishing the story" involves reminiscence for the sake of self in the present, heading into the future. It is very much a process of reading and rereading one's internal cognitive maps of values, beliefs, and meanings in order to develop a travel plan for the future.

If the process of aging presents a challenge to our sense of identity and integrity, then the confrontation with illness or injury only serves to potentiate the crisis. While the experience of illness or injury heightens the sense of mortality, admission to the hospital punctuates the vulnerability in terms of loss of independence and alienation from a more familiar life context.

A critical issue is whether the person possesses the inner resources to face the challenge. The trauma of illness, subsequent hospitalization, and recovery can represent a potentiation of the growth possibilities inherent in this life stage or simply a negation of the person and all that was held dear. The outcome depends upon the person's capacity to appropriate the experience of illness within some meaning-filled apprehension of himself or herself in relation to

his or her life story (Burghardt, 1991; Heinz, 1994).

Some individuals have found the discourse of faith and participation in a religious community meaningful in the past. They frequently present their coping response to the challenges of aging and illness in the actuation of a deeper spiritual awareness. This awareness, in turn, liberates much-needed psychological energy and resources. The discourse of psychology and rehabilitation may be meaningful to the provider of services and offers a liberating language to those persons who have been deeply alienated from religious communities. On the other hand, religious symbols, values, and meanings continue to provide a rich personal, interpersonal, and transpersonal narrative context within which many persons begin to construct or reconstruct the story of their lives.

However, as the faith development theorists (e.g., Fowler, 1981; Fowler et al., 1991) have brought to our attention, the language of faith of any given individual is not contained in some personal cookbook of cosmic remedies—easy and authoritative answers for life's dilemmas. Rather, the faith perspective changes and evolves as it is used to discern and comprehend life experiences. That process of transformation, subjectively considered, often creates significant uncertainty and doubt. Yet, descent into the "dark night of the soul," in which the person feels bereft of consolation, may mark a passage to a new faithful apprehension of self and world and subsequent mobilization of new capacities for coping.

BEYOND SUFFERING: REORGANIZING SENSE OF SELF AND RELATIONSHIPS IN THE LANGUAGE OF FAITH

A constructive developmental perspective on faith experience as a motivational factor in the process of rehabilitation, then, invites consideration of the specific manner in which individuals employ and rework religious beliefs, meanings, and values in order to reconstitute sense of self and sense of relatedness to others as the foundation of new motivational patterns. In order to unpack and illuminate this reconstructive process, I will offer case vignettes from my experiences as a chaplain to psychogeriatric patients over the past decade. Names and identifying data are either changed or deleted—their efforts to wrestle with Jacob's dark angel are presented with as much integrity and reverence as my words can muster.

The problem of evil and suffering has perplexed no less than Iraeneus, Augustine, Moses Maimonides, and Spinoza and finds us wondering still along with Rabbi Kushner (1981), "Why do bad things happen to good people?" The weight of this question falls as well on the elderly psychiatric patients with whom I have worked over the years. The generation of a constructive response to the suffering in their lives is very often the foundation upon which they begin to reconstruct their sense of self and community.

The onset of a severe psychiatric episode or the exacerbation of a dementing process presents a difficult challenge. Recovery invariably requires significant changes in habitual ways of living, beginning with compromise of independence and uprooting from familial and social networks. In the elderly, this scenario is often further complicated by physical disability or illness.

Patients are often admitted to the hospital in a sort of numb terror, which frequently begins to dissipate in the form of protest against their condition and circumstance—a protest that takes the form of the question, "Why has this happened to me? Why has God allowed this misery to come my way?"

When the question of suffering is raised by these patients it is often dismissed by clinicians oversocialized into the "zeitgeist" of modern health care professions as a defensive preoccupation. The patient's religious struggle may be diagnosed as mere hyperreligiosity associated with temporal lobe epilepsy, bipolar disorder, or subacute mood swings. But well after the antipsychotic medications, mood stabilizers, and/or antidepressants have loosened the grip of their symptoms, the question tends to persist, particularly for those patients with an established religious identification. That is only because, more often than not, this "human, all too human" question is the crucible for internal transformation. The question is not posed by their illness but by the humanity they share with all of us.

Lipowski (1970) has suggested that illness can be interpreted in eight ways: a challenge, an enemy, a punishment, a personal weakness, a relief, a strategy, an irreparable loss or damage, or a value. While Lipowski presents these interpretations of suffering as distinct positions, my general experience has been that they represent emerging perspectives on the issue of suffering within a process of meaningful adjustment. In other words, each position represents an understanding of the meaning of suffering that corresponds to the perspective shifts that occur as people progress from crisis to adjustment in constructing the meaning of who they are in relation to their suffering.

CASE STUDY 1

Recently, Mr. B., a 67-year-old, single, Protestant male with a history of bipolar disorder in relatively good control until the past several years, was admitted to the psychogeriatric unit in an acute manic phase exacerbated by alcohol abuse. His case was complicated by increased physical debility, which raised concerns regarding the onset of infarct dementia.

He had been living alone in the family home; his parents, with whom he had lived, had died several years earlier. Since his parents' death, he had frequent exacerbations of his illness and multiple hospitalizations because he had gone off his medications and had begun drinking heavily. Collaterals informed the social worker that he had become progressively disorganized recently, seeming more and more incapable of caring for himself and managing the home.

He angrily and vehemently denied any problems and righteously admonished the staff that he was the "Chosen One of Israel." Even after he was detox-

ified and the mood stabilizers had reduced his symptoms, he presented as resistant to assessments and interventions focusing on his rehabilitation. He did so with a certain righteous indignation that seemed more related to the narcissistic insult occasioned by his illness and hospitalization.

At the time of admission Mr. B. had self-identified as Protestant and was interested in pastoral visitation. In the beginning the intensity of his symptoms prevented anything more that brief visits for the purpose of gathering basic information regarding his religious background and practice prior to hospitalization. I learned that he had attended church regularly though somewhat more sporadically after his parents' death and often read the Bible. This suggested to me that religious interests were likely a significant component of his life context and not simply related to the exacerbation of his illness.

As his symptoms began to subside and Mr. B. became somewhat more available, he was able to express to me what appeared to be the core issue— a fundamentally spiritual one—in his struggle to accept treatment at this point in time. He informed me that he had always been fascinated by the story of the "Prodigal Son." He pointed out that his stronger identification had always been with the elder son, whom he perceived as the "good son" who did not squander his portion of the inheritance. In fact, being the "good son" was at the heart of his personal narrative, striving to please a father whom he idealized despite describing a father who had physically and emotionally abused him as a child and derided him for his illness as an adult.

From this initial perspective his movement into suffering could only be viewed as something extrinsic and foreign to the fundamental organization of his personal identity and destiny. To acknowledge the need for treatment would be to acknowledge the presence of vulnerability and weakness, which his overidentification with the "good son" could not allow.

Even as he shared his story of the good son and the merciless father, a certain disengagement from this identification began to occur. Confronted by his treaters with the likely prospect that he would not be returning to the family home soon, if ever, the foundations of his personal myth were being shaken.

He shared with me in one visit, "Perhaps I am more like the prodigal son than I care to admit. I'm losing my inheritance and nothing can save me." At this phase of his crisis he became severely depressed and his resistance to treatment stiffened. If he seemed to be regressing, however, it was only in the interests of health for, in fact, his construction of the crisis had changed. He had begun to acknowledge that the crisis was somehow related to himself as an internal datum and not simply some foreign attribution forced upon him by his treaters.

This interim passage in his journey began with a shift in perspective as the illness became an internal reality, though experienced as a punishment for past sins and indiscretions, not least of which was never having really lived up to his father's expectations. Here it was absolutely critical to accept and help him explore the intense anger and rage that he felt, first toward God and then toward his father, as he moved beyond his denial of his illness and himself. The rage and anger were prompted by a valuation of his identification with the prodigal son from the perspective of the good son. However, as his identification with the prodigal son deepened and we considered the narrative for what seemed like the millionth time, he began to see that the prodigal son is not rejected. In fact, he is not even judged despite having squandered half the family inheritance. Rather, he is accepted, embraced, and reinstated, though this time with a capacity to accept his own vulnerability. He seemed to be discovering, as the narrative thrust of the story goes, that the suffering of the prodigal son is not punishment but the occasion for discovering something new in his relationship to the father—the father's capacity for acceptance—something the good son never sees or understands.

The stance toward suffering by the end of the narrative, both in the story of the prodigal son and Mr. B., is a movement beyond despair toward integrity, in which suffering, without value of its own, is and should be accepted only insofar as it serves the vocation of the second half of life—fuller self-acceptance.

The relevance of Mr. B.'s inner journey in the broader context of his rehabilitation emerged for me in observing a parallel process in which his denial and resistance for treatment gradually shifted toward an ability to engage in and use the interventions offered to him by various rehabilitation specialists. Expressed in religious terms, he had moved toward an answer to the motivational question that was blocking his treatment, "Does the acceptance of suffering as an aspect of who I am constitute a movement toward integrity or a capitulation to despair?"

In Mr. B.'s case, the medium of transformation was an inward journey consisting of self-examination guided by a religious narrative uniquely powerful for him at this time in his life—such an inward spiritual negotiation of the crisis of integrity was a process consistent with his pietistic Protestant religious background. However, religiosity is expressed with subsequent attitudinal transformations occurring in a variety of ways, not the least of which is through the more action-oriented process of ritual performance and practice.

CASE STUDY 2

Judaism, like Christianity, not to mention other world religions, has its contemplative, reflective side and that aspect that is more focused on the expression of faith through ritual observance and practice. Ms. R.'s case illustrates the manner in which the engagement in a religious practice served to mediate and reconstitute a sense of connectedness that, in turn, seemed to enable her to gather together her resources to face the tasks of rehabilitation.

Ms. R. was a 69-year-old, widowed, Jewish woman who was admitted to the psychogeriatric unit appearing withdrawn, disorganized, and apparently unable to care for herself. Following

consultation with collaterals who reported increased isolation, paranoia, and disorganization during her slow recovery from a hip fracture, diagnostic possibilities considered were senile dementia and/or major depression with psychotic features.

Her psychosocial profile indicated that she had been married for 34 years and that her husband had died 10 years before. Since then she had been living alone. The couple had a daughter, now married and living on the West Coast, who visited two or three times a year. She also had three sisters and two brothers, one of whom was in a nursing home in New York. She had had no significant contact with any of them for several years and had not been close to anyone in her family since she was married, per her report. In fact, her family made efforts to contact her that she dismissed and resisted in the early phase of her hospitalization. Her record noted that social supports had deteriorated over the past 10 years due to her increasing isolation and now consisted primarily of part-time home-care nurses.

In the course of a pastoral services needs assessment, which I conducted with her, she self-identified as a nonpracticing Jew. Her husband, she reported, had been Protestant. Neither partner had actively practiced any religion in many years. She indicated that she was not interested in pastoral services at that time.

Subsequent notations in her record indicated that she responded relatively well to a course of neuroleptics and antidepressants. Some symptom reduction was observed but Ms. R. remained isolative and diffident about her participation in rehabilitation treatment. She would occasionally attend groups and engage in physical therapy related to recovery from the hip fracture. She often complained, however, of being too tired to get involved in anything. Staff observed her sitting and dozing in a corner of the day hall or in her room, when she could get away with it.

She had been hospitalized for several months when news came that her brother in the nursing home was dying. When informed of this, Ms. R. insisted that she be allowed to attend his funeral. After struggling with this, the treatment team reached the decision to allow her to attend. However, the brother died much sooner than expected, which prevented appropriate arrangements from being made. Ms. R. was absolutely overcome with anger and grief. The staff called me to come and see her, as she had, for the first time, requested to see a chaplain— in her words, "Preferably the Jewish chaplain, but one of the others will have to do."

As I was the chaplain on call, I went to see her, intrigued by her unexpected request. After informing me in the first few minutes of the visit of her brother's death, she broke into tears and said, "I must say Kaddish for him, but I no longer remember the prayer ... only that I need a candle"; and then she cried for a few minutes. "Fortunately," I told her, "we have a rabbi who can help us." Arrangements were made with the rabbi and several Jewish staff members to meet with the woman at the appointed hour and say Kaddish with her.

Her interest in continuing to meet with the rabbi led to regularly scheduled visits that resulted, as I observed, in a revitalized interest in and identification with a religious heritage that she had forsaken in early adulthood. This interest was paralleled by an exploration of the impact of the many losses in her life. The sequelae of this reconstitution of her religious identity was a renewed interest in contact with her family and a willingness to participate in rehabilitative treatment, which eventually made it possible to discharge her to a rest home in New York near other members of her family.

In reference to the problem of her own suffering, her practice of the rite appears to have mediated a fundamentally different stance with respect to the suffering in her own life marked by the loss of her husband, the loss of her brother, and, longer ago, the loss of a fundamental part of herself. Her performance of the ritual of the Kaddish, the Jewish prayer of mourning, marked an acknowledgment of the suffering in her life as her own, and an act whereby she defined the suffering rather than allowing it to define her.

A CONCLUDING SEMI-SCIENTIFIC POSTSCRIPT

I have worked side by side with scientifically trained clinicians in psychiatric settings for many years. My general observation is that they are more attuned to contraindications for integration of the patient's religious interests into treatment than they are to consideration of its constructive potential.

A certain caution is understandable, particularly in psychiatric settings. Clinicians are often confronted with the more glaring contraindications, such as when a patient's religious interests are clearly delusional or obsessional, are rooted in sociopathy (the Elmer Gantry syndrome), or are intertwined with defensive structures associated with severe personality disorders.

But the extent to which the inner life has been neglected as a critical component in the rehabilitation process bespeaks the extent to which rehabilitation disciplines have relied upon an objectivist stance. Perhaps this stance reflects their desire to speak the language of hard science even when their intention is to attend to the reality of individuals not simply as complexes of factors, functions, and processes but as living, intending, meaning-making persons.

In short, there is much work to be done in terms of building the bridges between religion and rehabilitation, a task that requires the efforts of "hard" *and* "soft" science. A number of more empirically oriented research efforts certainly commend continued exploration of the positive role of faith and religion in the rehabilitation process. At this time substantial research supports a high correlation among physical health, sense of well-being, and active connection with a religious/faith tradition across the life span (Spilka, Hood, & Gorsuch, 1985). Even more significant, the growing research in "mind/body medicine" (Benson, 1975; Borysenko, 1988; Kabat-Zinn, 1990) is documenting an increasingly clear connection

and positive correlation between a vital inner life and biophysical as well as psychosocial integrity.

The tendency, however, of such research is to establish correlations from an objectivist standpoint that trade in statistical probabilities, when the more fundamental work of rehabilitation is to relate to the concrete presence of a person. Thus, phenomenological approaches, which rely on "thick description" of the transformative processes from the standpoint of the subject, will be critical in amplifying the "meaningful" integration of biophysical, psychological, social, and spiritual dimensions of the healing process. Recognition of the relevance of "life contexts" and "volitional narratives" in the rehabilitation process represents a significant movement in the direction of a holistic method, which is more adequate to the complexity of motivation and the fullness of being human.

REFERENCES

Bateson, G. (1956). Communication in occupational therapy. *American Journal of Occupational Therapy, 10,* 188.

Benson, H. (1975). *The relaxation response.* New York: Morrow.

Borysenko, J. (1988). *Minding the body: Mending the mind.* New York: Bantam Books.

Burghardt, W. (1991). Aging, suffering and dying: A Christian perspective. In L.S. Cahill & D. Mieth (Eds.), *Aging.* London: Trinity Press International.

Englehardt, H.T., Jr. (1977). Defining occupational therapy: The meaning of therapy and the virtues of occupation. *American Journal of Occupational Therapy, 31,* 666–672.

Erikson, E. (1950). *Childhood and society.* New York: Norton.

Fowler, J. (1981). *Stages of faith.* San Francisco: Harper & Row.

Fowler, J., Nipkow, K., & Schweitzer, F. (Eds.). (1991). *Stages of faith and religious development.* New York: Crossroads.

Heinz, D. (1994). Finishing the story: Aging, spirituality and the work of culture. *Journal of Religious Gerontology, 9*(1), 3–19.

Helfrich, C., & Kielhofner, G. (1994). Volitional narratives and the meaning of therapy. *American Journal of Occupational Therapy, 48,* 319–326.

Kabat-Zinn, J. (1990). *Full catastrophe living.* New York: Dell.

Kegan, R. (1980). There the dance is: Religious dimensions of developmental theory. In C. Brusselmans, J. Fowler, J. O'Donohoe, & Y. A. Vergote (Eds.), *Toward moral and religious maturity.* Morristown, NJ: Silver Burdett.

Kegan, R. (1983). *The evolving self.* Cambridge, MA: Harvard University Press.

Kegan, R. (1994). *In over our heads.* Cambridge, MA: Harvard University Press.

Kushner, H. (1981). *When bad things happen to good people.* New York: Avon Books.

Lipowski, Z.J. (1970). Physical illness, the individual and the coping process. *International Journal of Psychiatry and Medicine, 1,* 91–102.

McDargh, J. (1983). *Psychoanalytic object relations theory and the study of religion: On faith and the imaging of God.* Lanham, MD: University Press of America.

Rosenfeld, M. (1993). *Wellness and lifestyle renewal: A manual for personal change.* Bethesda, MD: American Occupational Therapy Association.

Spilka, B., Hood, R., & Gorsuch, L. (1985). *The psychology of religion: An empirical approach.* Englewood Cliffs, NJ: Prentice-Hall.

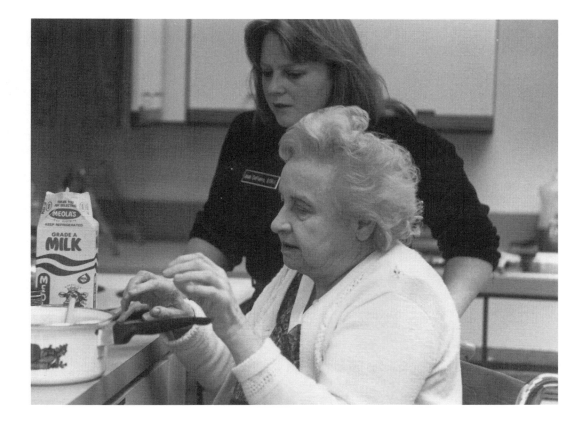

12 *Evaluating Motivation and Rehabilitation Potential*

Robert R. Read, EdD and Mark S. Rosenfeld, PhD, OTR/L

The case vignettes presented in this book illuminate the importance of patient motivation in geriatric rehabilitation. This chapter examines the literature pertaining to assessment of patient motivation, discusses the absence of any instruments to assess or measure motivation, and presents suggestions of formats and instruments for aiding in such assessments. Finally a "Measure of Subacute Rehabilitation Potential" devised by the editor is presented and demonstrated using case material.

The importance of assessing patient motivation as part of an evaluation of rehabilitation potential is mentioned repeatedly in the occupational therapy literature (Bonder, 1992; Brummell-Smith, 1993; Kemp, 1990; Versluys, 1995). Holistic or integrative approaches to patient care maintain that biological, social, and psychological domains of the individual should be considered in evaluation and treatment planning (Hemphill, 1988; Joseph & Wanlass, 1993; Mosqueda, 1993). Motivation is placed in the psychological domain and is viewed problematically as illusive, poorly defined, difficult to quantify or specify, and in need of further clarification, codification, and research (Kemp, 1990); concomitantly it is also acknowledged as an essential, pivotal ingredient in positive patient prognosis and treatment outcome (Helfrich, Kielhofner, & Mattingly, 1994; Kemp, 1990). How ironic, then, that no objective instruments for accurate, empirical, or efficient assessment of motivation exist.

A review of occupational therapy literature yielded no instruments constructed for the assessment of motivation. For example, in *Mental Health Assessments in Occupational Therapy* (Hemphill, 1988) there is no index listing for motivation and only one mention of it in the entire text. Personal discussions with senior occupational therapists and directors of geriatric settings similarly produced no evidence that such assessment tools exist, despite the fact that these seasoned clinicians acknowledged the critical importance of motivation in rehabilitation.

Because motivation is a psychological construct, the psychological literature was also examined for assessment instruments. The citations under motivation in *The Eleventh Mental Measures*

Yearbook (Kramer & Conoley, 1992), the "bible" of psychological tests and measures, were focused primarily on student achievement and motivation. There were no measures associated with rehabilitation potential, geriatric settings, or the elderly. A new text focusing specifically on presenting and synthesizing the findings of assessment instruments pertaining to medical rehabilitation (Cushman & Scherer, 1995) includes no instruments related to motivation. Discussions with geriatric psychologists, nursing home psychologists, and researchers again yielded no relevant measures but did produce additional confirmation based on their experiences of the importance of motivation for successful rehabilitation. Psychological literature on motivation from related disciplines argues the critical importance of motivation in all processes of change or growth (Miller & Rollnick, 1991), but that literature offers no instruments for objective assessment.

We are therefore left with a paradoxical situation. The importance of motivation seems well-established by research, theory, and clinical experience, yet there are no empirical measures to assess it. Experience gives health care practitioners keen appreciation of the importance of the patient's motivation or lack thereof, and they thus assess it intuitively during the clinical interview or amid interaction with the patient. Such impressionistic approaches to assessment of patient motivation are important but vulnerable to clinician bias and to possible failure to appreciate differences in what motivates people (Neistadt, 1995; Ramsden, 1988). The case vignettes in this book illustrate the centrality of motivation in rehabilitation potential. Research and clinical practice endorse its importance. Clearly an effort to present assessment heuristics, strategies, and instruments is warranted.

RELATIONAL CONTEXT FOR ASSESSMENT

Current approaches to patient care in all medical disciplines are guided by the interrelated elements of *collaboration* (Neistadt, 1995; Ramsden, 1988; Thibodaux & Shewchuk, 1988) and the recognized importance of the patient–clinician *relationship* (Fleury, 1991; Schunk, 1988). Treatment outcome, patient motivation, compliance with treatment, and prognosis are increasingly recognized as significantly affected by inclusion of the patient in the treatment planning process and, in part via such inclusion, by having a relationship with those involved in the treatment. Thus assessment of patient motivation for rehabilitation should take place in a consciously forged collaborative relationship with the patient. Establishing this context, called "joining" or "creating rapport" in the psychological domain, is often done intuitively by occupational therapists during the initial clinical interview with patients.

SUBJECTIVE ASSESSMENT

Consciously joining with the patient and inquiring curiously about the patient's former work or interests begins to establish a working relationship while gathering data relevant to understanding the patient's world. Functional assessments about activities of daily living are not sufficient to understand a patient and how he or she is reacting to disability and possible rehabilitation. After all, how can we understand a patient to enable him or her to engage in a treatment regime if we do not understand what the disability means to the patient, what has been lost, what is to be gained? Recalling Kemp's (1990) definition of motivation as described by Rosenfeld in chapter 2 of this book, we must explore with the patient his or her existential perception of losses, costs, and gains in relation to rewards to begin to understand and assess the patient's motivation.

Kemp (1990) neatly conceptualizes motivation in a formula that can guide the practitioner in formulating an understanding of the patient's level of motivation.

$$\text{Motivation} = \frac{\text{Wants} \times \text{Beliefs} \times \text{Rewards}}{\text{Costs}}$$

In Kemp's formula *wants* include desires, wishes, needs, and goals; *beliefs* include assumptions and perceptions; and *rewards* include reinforcements and benefits. *Costs* are the perceived negative consequences or risks. Kemp is careful to point out the highly subjective nature of motivation and therefore emphasizes the centrality of collaborative treatment planning and abundant rewards. This theoretical formula of assessing motivation can be a helpful guide to the clinician in goal setting and treatment planning.

The clinical interview establishes the collaborative relationship from which to set goals with the patient. These goals

derive from psychosocial information obtained in the interview. It makes more sense to devise a treatment program using an activity known and loved by the patient than one using an activity unrelated to their interests or future needs. This goal setting, intimately related to hearing the patient's narrative as described above, should be considered an *intervention*, geared toward gathering relevant treatment planning information while forming a collaborative relationship with the patient.

Such an exploration also must be historical, taking into consideration aspects of the patient's life that may have bearing on motivation. Thus in the relationship-building, collaborative interview, an effort should be made to begin eliciting and hearing what Helfrich et al. (1994) call the patient's "narrative," or the story of what has been important in a patient's life. Contemporary motivational theory (Miller & Rollnick, 1991; Prochaska & DiClemente, 1986) argues the importance in any change process of accurately determining where the individual is in terms of his or her readiness for change. Establishing a collaboration in the context of a relationship and hearing the patient's narrative to determine what has been important to this patient, what has motivated him or her in the past, what he or she has done that was meaningful or inspiring—these help the clinician begin to determine where the patient is in terms of readiness to change (in this context to deal with disability and a program of rehabilitation) and to listen for or elicit information pertinent to establishing mutually determined treatment goals and strategies to attain them.

OBJECTIVE ASSESSMENT INSTRUMENTS

The informal, diagnostic interview is an essential but insufficient part of assessing patient motivation for rehabilitation. Fast-paced clinical practice combined with reimbursement issues are in direct conflict with the relational, more subjective aspects of clinical practice emphasized in much of the literature. Hence, practitioners must attend to both areas by more thoughtfully using the clinical interview and by using more empirical instruments in their assessments.

Mini Mental Status Exam (MMSE)

A motivational *assessment* should be considered part of a motivational *intervention*. Interactional discussion with a patient about what has been important in the past and what is important in the future is a form of data gathering to assemble with the patient goals and a treatment plan emanating from them. In the context of this interview, the clinician should be listening carefully to the patient for signs of depression or cognitive impairment. Depression and cognitive impairment affect a significant percentage of geriatric patients and negatively affect motivation. If any signs of such problems are present, a Mini Mental Status Exam (Folstein, Folstein, & McHugh, 1975) can be integrated verbally into the interview. The MMSE is short, easily administered and scored, and has been researched for validity and reliability. If the MMSE scores indicate

that a patient is depressed or cognitively impaired, it is reasonable to assume that motivation will be negatively affected. Assessment will now have an objective dimension and the initial treatment plan should include steps to address the motivational problems.

Measure of Subacute Rehabilitation Potential (MOSARP)

As noted above, the informal interview is insufficient because it is too susceptible to clinician bias. Rosenfeld (1994) has devised a more objective instrument, the *Measure of Subacute Rehabilitation Potential* (see Figure 1), which can be briefly and easily filled out and scored as part of the diagnostic interview. Rosenfeld has constructed this measure based on distilling and combining key factors in positive prognosis for rehabilitation gleaned from the literature. The instrument consists of 20 items that address the main areas of health status, history, hope, help, and health efforts. Clinicians assess a patient by rating each item on a Likert scale from 1 (a very negative factor in rehabilitation potential) to 5 (a very positive factor in rehabilitation potential). These items have been found to have construct validity in two pilot studies (Breidel et al., 1996; Van Etten, 1995). These studies yielded high agreement between health care clinicians, patients, and healthy adults, who rated as most important to rehabilitation potential the ability to participate in treatment and rely on a treatment team. (Interestingly, the Breidel study also found that the more veteran a clinician, the less importance he or she placed on medication, current health

FIGURE 1. MEASURE OF SUBACUTE REHABILITATION POTENTIAL

The following five categories list factors that positively influence rehabilitation potential. To establish a patient's level of readiness for occupational therapy treatment, rate each factor from 1–5 in the spaces provided. A rating of 5 indicates a very positive factor; 3 indicates a balance of positive and negative influences. A rating of 1 indicates a very negative factor. Add the ratings for all 20 items to compute a summary score for the individual. In using the summary scores below, please recognize that treatment may be justified in some instances, despite a low score, because of the importance of a single factor or cluster of factors.

Scores range as follows: 20–39 = very low rehabilitation potential
40–59 = low–moderate rehabilitation potential
60–79 = high–moderate rehabilitation potential
80–100 = very high rehabilitation potential

Health Status	Age a positive factor (closer to 60 than 90)	_____
	Mild diagnostic profile	_____
	Effective treatment options	_____
	Positive general prognosis	_____
History	Of handling pain, loss, or anxiety well	_____
	Of confronting and surmounting crisis	_____
	Of defining and accepting challenge	_____
	Of meaningful life and occupations	_____
Hope	For continued life or meaning in death	_____
	For healing and recovery	_____
	For improved functioning, quality of life	_____
	For positive living environment	_____
Help	Available supports (material, medical, social)	_____
	Relatedness and acceptance of support	_____
	Response to dependency status	_____
	Ability to collaborate and communicate needs	_____
Health Efforts	Psychic and physical energy	_____
	Goal clarity and adoption, cognitive skills	_____
	Task performance skills, follow-through	_____
	Outcome performance appraisal	_____
	Total	_____

Summary:

condition, and prognosis. This finding suggests further support for the importance of psychosocial factors, including the collaborative treatment relationship, in overall treatment outcome.) Interrater reliability studies are currently under way. Further development and study are required before summary ratings produced by the instrument can be used with confidence; nonetheless, this tool offers the first systematic vehicle for the holistic evaluation of factors influencing rehabilitation potential. The next section includes instructions for its clinical use, followed by a detailed case illustration.

GUIDELINES FOR USING THE MOSARP

MOSARP should be used in conjunction with functional evaluation. Therapists typically assess premorbid functioning, current mobility skills, strength, range of motion, coordination, endurance, cognition, ADL skills, and safety awareness. Occupational roles, interests, and goals are of major importance along with the characteristics and functional requirements of the proposed discharge environment.

Data relevant for MOSARP ratings are gathered through chart review; interviews with the patient, significant others, and interdisciplinary staff members; and the therapist's direct observation of patient responses. Time spent with the individual offers the therapist opportunities to observe how the patient responds to illness and pain; to communicate about the future; and to offer assistance with immediate, practical problems and tasks.

The 20 items included in the measure cue the therapist to seek specific information from and about the patient. Many of the items can be assessed by asking direct questions. In the *history* section, for example, it is useful to ask the patient and family members about previous hardships in the patient's life. What challenges and adversities has the individual experienced? How well did the patient cope with his or her feelings? How did the patient tackle the problems he or she faced?

Direct interview is also effective in evaluating the *hope* category. What expectations does the patient have for the future? What beliefs are held about illness and about the prospects for treatment and recovery? Where does the person hope to live? When patients say they want to go home, therapists should ask, "What are you looking forward to doing when you get there?"

Ratings are made for the 20 items based on the therapists's clinical judgment of the extent to which each one positively or negatively influences the effective rehabilitation effort on the part of the patient. Norms for summary scores are not yet developed. Therefore, these summary scores yield only an impression of high, moderate, or low rehabilitation potential when viewed in context of other evaluation results. In addition, treatment potential may be quite stable for some patients, while it may be rather fluid and subject to changing events, circumstances, time, and relationships with others.

Individual ratings can be of critical importance, therefore, in identifying specific areas that will support or weaken the patient's involvement in the rehabilitation program. While two areas—health status and history—are beyond alteration, the patient's behavior patterns related to hope, help, and health efforts may be influenced through therapeutic interventions.

Even historical factors can be improved on. Despite a poor history of handling adversity and of occupational satisfaction, for example, gains can still be made through new attitudes, strategies, and skills. If patients are unrealistically negative in their hopes for the future, information, reality testing, problem solving, and modeling by other patients can frequently turn the tide.

While available resources may be fixed, items in the *help* category may clearly be influenced as well. Therapists can certainly support and instruct caregivers. They can foster improved communication and collaboration through therapeutic contact and encourage patients to accept assistance or to strive harder for independence as needed.

Finally, *health efforts* can be strengthened in a number of ways. Prescriptions can be sought for medications to decrease depression, anxiety, or pain, and thereby improve energy available for treatment activities. Careful discussion and planning can lead to adoption of clear goals that mobilize patients to work hard in treatment. Therapists can also help patients to make realistic appraisals of their performance and progress.

Based on evaluation results, a summary note is written at the bottom of the MOSARP form that defines the patient's current treatment potential, identifies pivotal areas of strength and

weakness, and makes a program recommendation. The therapist may suggest that treatment begin; that treatment is not viable at this time; or that specific, time-limited measures be attempted to improve rehabilitation potential.

CASE EXAMPLE USING THE MOSARP

The following case illustrates the assessment of rehabilitation potential and the motivational interventions to improve it.

Ann, a 71-year-old widow, status post CVA and with a long history of hospitalization for manic depressive illness, was admitted to a nursing home for rehabilitation after discharge from an acute inpatient medical unit. The patient had incurred a fractured sternum when her husband suffered a heart attack and crashed the car. Husband died at the scene, and the patient was transported by ambulance to the hospital. Three days later, medically stable, Ann was transferred to the subacute facility.

For 7 days she sat in a darkened room, wrapped in a blanket, allowing only minimal nursing care for vital signs, toileting, and meals. When rehabilitation staff entered her room to conduct evaluations, Ann screamed at them to get out and leave her alone. The therapists understood her reasons for being angry and upset. They also felt intimidated by the intensity of her screams and verbal threats. As of the seventh day of her stay, Ann had refused all attempts at evaluation. The rehabilitation manager predicted that she would be decertified for skilled services in the Medicare meeting later that day due to persistent noncompliance.

As a per diem occupational therapist with a strong mental health background, I was asked to give Ann one last try. Recognizing that this patient was in crisis and coping poorly with overwhelming feelings, I planned to tackle emotional issues immediately. I knocked, stepped in, and introduced myself as an occupational therapist. I stated that I would not let her throw me out, and that she and I would talk that morning. "Why the hell should I talk to you?" she shouted. "Because you are suffering terribly because of what's happened. You have to let someone get his shoulder under this burden with you. You need some support."

Ann began to cry softly. I pulled up a chair and sat down. I mentioned that I had met her psychiatrist. "He stinks!" she said vehemently. "You mean treatment never really helped your depression?" I asked. "No. Medicine and ECT never helped," Ann lamented.

"Has life been a complete misery then?" I inquired. Ann admitted that raising her two children had been a real joy, and that her husband was a good companion. She burst into tears then, and I helped her dry her eyes with some tissues. Then I asked about the accident and her husband's death. Ann told the story in painful detail. The events had been sudden and overwhelming. She never saw her husband again after the accident and could not even attend the funeral due to her own injury and hospitalization. "No wonder you've been hiding in here." I commented. "You can't face the world again until you have had a chance to grieve."

"I don't know where in the world I belong now," Ann declared. "My daughter asked me to live with her and her kids. But I'm so helpless, I can't even dress myself. I relied so much on my husband since my stroke. He even brushed my teeth for me. How could I live with my daughter? I love her and the kids, but I'd be like another child to take care of. Maybe I should just stay in the nursing home." This subject cued me to introduce the idea of occupational therapy evaluation and treatment. "Well," I said, "let's see what you can do. If I help you to do more for yourself, then you will be on stronger ground when it is time to decide where to live." "Right now I need to go to the bathroom," Ann stated. "Then let's see how you can get there using your cane," I suggested. Functional evaluation proceeded. Based on her mobility, strength, and cognitive performance on several ADL tasks, it became clear that this patient could benefit from occupational therapy treatment.

Toward the end of this first session, I told Ann that grief and tears can last a year following a spouse's death. I stressed that she must continue to talk, cry, and accept support about this loss. I reminded her that she was not really very old and that she should eventually find some ways to enjoy life, perhaps more fully than she had before. "And do more for myself again," she added. "Yes," I agreed, "and you have made a good start on that today!"

Following this session and a discussion with Ann's daughter, I completed the Measure of Subacute Rehabilitation Potential (see Figure 2). The ratings

FIGURE 2. MEASURE OF SUBACUTE REHABILITATION POTENTIAL

Ann, 12/1/94

The following five categories list factors that positively influence rehabilitation potential. To establish a patient's level of readiness for occupational therapy treatment, rate each factor from 1–5 in the spaces provided. A rating of 5 indicates a very positive factor; 3 indicates a balance of positive and negative influences. A rating of 1 indicates a very negative factor. Add the ratings for all 20 items to compute a summary score for the individual. In using the summary scores below, please recognize that treatment may be justified in some instances, despite a low score, because of the importance of a single factor or cluster of factors.

Scores range as follows: 20–39 = very low rehabilitation potential
40–59 = low–moderate rehabilitation potential
60–79 = high–moderate rehabilitation potential
80–100 = very high rehabilitation potential

Health Status	Age a positive factor (closer to 60 than 90)	5
	Mild diagnostic profile	3
	Effective treatment options	5
	Positive general prognosis	3
History	Of handling pain, loss, or anxiety well	1
	Of confronting and surmounting crisis	1
	Of defining and accepting challenge	1
	Of meaningful life and occupations	1
Hope	For continued life or meaning in death	2
	For healing and recovery	2
	For improved functioning, quality of life	3
	For positive living environment	4
Help	Available supports (material, medical, social)	5
	Relatedness and acceptance of support	3
	Response to dependency status	1
	Ability to collaborate and communicate needs	2
Health Efforts	Psychic and physical energy	3
	Goal clarity and adoption, cognitive skills	2
	Task performance skills, follow-through	2
	Outcome performance appraisal	3
	Total	52

Summary: Low–Moderate Rehabilitation Potential

This pt's medical condition, age (71), and supportive children are relatively positive factors. History of poor crisis-meeting resources and tendency to adopt hostile-dependent stance are major deterrents to effective treatment. Recommend approach offering strong support for expression of grief re death of husband, identification of future living options, and life goals. Tie goals to pt's efforts to work with OTs and increase ADL performance, adopt active-coping orientation, and express and manage grief.

Mark S. Rosenfeld, PhD, OTR/L

helped to define and clarify the positive and negative factors influencing Ann's participation in treatment and to justify her continued approval for skilled services. The following describes my ratings and my thinking in each area of the evaluation. A "5" is the most positive and a "1" the most negative rating for each item.

Health status is a mildly positive area for this patient. At age 71, Ann is in the "young elderly" category. Her previous stroke had created mild to moderate weakness and disability on the nondominant side. No perceptual, cognitive, or communication problems were noted. The fractured sternum was healing well. No traumatic organ damage was reported. Manic depressive illness had been quite debilitating, however, with a chronic course. Occupational therapy methods to improve mobility, safety, and ADL skills (the patient's stated goals) were plentiful. Graded task assignments are frequently effective in overcoming the passivity, psychomotor retardation, and negative self-assessment associated with depression. Considering both medical and psychiatric conditions, Ann's overall prognosis appeared fair.

History is an area of significant weakness. The patient's initial response to traumatic loss was maladaptive. She had retreated to a profound level of dependency following her stroke 5 years previous. Bipolar disorder contributed to Ann's tendency to become discouraged and helpless under duress. She perceived the threat and loss in crisis events but not the challenge. Therefore, she had failed to mobilize an active coping response in the past and had not tackled rehabilitation tasks well following her stroke. Ann also experienced little success in surmounting her psychiatric symptoms. She felt negatively about her quality of life, despite valued family relationships and success in raising two children. She reported only mild former interests in Bingo and board games.

Hope was an area of mixed influences. Ann believed she would continue to live but had low expectations for her quality of life. While she knew that her sternum would heal, Ann did not think that she would overcome her persistent depression, her dependency, or the traumatic loss of her husband. She was tentative about her ability to restore any functional skills now that her husband could no longer take care of her. Ironically, she associated dependency with a low quality of life, despite her entrenched passivity. More positively, Ann did associate improved functional skills with the possibility of living with or near her daughter and grandchildren. This desire served as a focus for the patient's tentative future aspirations.

Help was an important area, with some conflicting influences for Ann. The patient's daughter, son, and grandchildren were emotionally close and concerned, although they lived 2 hours from the facility. Daughter was genuine in her desire for mother to live with her family. Despite her complaints, Ann had a relationship with her psychiatrist spanning 15 years. The doctor reported that Ann frequently expressed appreciation for his help and concern. Material resources and health insurance were adequate to support needed rehabilitation, medical, and psychiatric services, as well as home care services, if necessary in the future. Ann certainly had a history of hostile-dependent behavior. While Ann had initially rejected help at the nursing home, she had communicated and collaborated well with the therapist once her overwhelming feelings were addressed. She subsequently engaged with other therapists and patients during an exercise group that same day.

Health efforts was an area of initial weakness but one with potential. Ann's psychic energy was absorbed by wrenching emotions related to the accident, injury, and spouse's death. Physical energy was low due to depression and deconditioning. Pain was a minor obstacle to rehabilitation effort. When ready, however, this patient demonstrated reasonable energy and effort in mobility evaluation and in the exercise group. Ann's cognitive skills were intact, although active problem solving was weak. She did not have any clear goals initially but understood the need to work toward a vision of a desired future. Ann's task performance skills were quite eroded. She tended to wait for others to do for her. She required constant cueing and supervision to initiate any task and to follow through. With cueing and support, however, she had made reasonable efforts in mobility and ADL tasks. Ann made only negative or neutral judgments about her performance during the evaluation. She was reluctant to make positive statements about her efforts but did genuinely accept praise from the therapist.

In summary, MOSARP results indicated that Ann's age, health status, and available supports were relatively positive factors. History of poor crisis-meeting resources and profound dependency presented obstacles to effective rehabilitation. In the context of her husband's death, Ann had also lost hope and direction for the future. Therefore, she had made no productive efforts and failed to work with the therapists assigned to her case.

In contrast to her dismal start at this facility, this patient was found to have moderate rehabilitation potential. This potential hinged on several factors: continued healthy grieving; active collaboration with rehabilitation staff; adoption of personal goals to improve ADL performance and demonstration of concerted efforts to do so; restoration of hope for purposeful, enjoyable use of time and for discharge to a desired living environment.

These issues were discussed with Ann, her children, and the rehabilitation staff. With clear nuclear tasks in mind, treatment proceeded smoothly. A scrapbook about her husband and regular Bingo participation were added to ADL and mobility training activities. Based on Kemp's (1990) equation for treatment motivation, it seemed that living with or near her daughter's family was the patient's "want" and a potential "reward" for rehabilitation efforts. "Beliefs" about herself as a permanently helpless burden were challenged by the therapist and by Ann's own observations as she tried and succeeded in treatment activities. The major "cost" involved the loss of secondary gains. Ann had received a great deal of nurturance in response to her infantile, dependent stance. Her husband's death removed the source of this nurturance. While this precipitated a crisis, it also created an opportunity for growth. Therapy became a vehicle for this growth by supporting expression and management of feelings along with concrete task challenges the patient could tackle.

Ann attended sessions consistently and worked hard. Before her discharge a month later, she admitted that she was amazed to realize how completely helpless she had allowed herself to become in her life. She transferred to a nursing home in New Hampshire to be near her daughter and grandchildren and expected to continue to work toward assisted living in a location near her family.

Rehabilitation success, in this case, depended on attention to motivational issues, application of crisis intervention methods, and systematic assessment of rehabilitation potential. Without such a holistic approach to evaluation, treatment compliance may have been compromised, and functional goals, quality of life, and reimbursement opportunities might have been lost.

REFERENCES

Bonder, B. (1992). Issues in assessment of the psychosocial component of function. *American Journal of Occupational Therapy, 47,* 211–216.

Breidel, D., Donoian, A.M., Landry, C., Parandes, K., Rock, D., Seiden, A., & Twarog, N. (1996). *A measure of rehab potential.* Unpublished paper.

Brummell-Smith, K. (1993). Research in rehabilitation. *Clinics in Geriatric Medicine, 9,* 895–904.

Cushman, L., & Scherer, M. (Eds.). (1995). *Psychological assessment in medical rehabilitation.* Washington, DC: American Psychological Association.

Fleury, J. (1991). Empowering potential: A theory of wellness motivation, *Nursing Research, 40,* 286–291.

Folstein, M.F., Folstein, S., & McHugh, P.R. (1975). Mini-mental state: A practical method for grading the cognitive state of patients for the clinician. *Journal of Psychiatric Residents, 12,* 189.

Joseph, C., & Wanlass, W. (1993). Rehabilitation in the nursing home. *Geriatric Rehabilitation, 9,* 859–871.

Helfrich, C., Kielhofner, G., & Mattingly, C. (1994). Volition as narrative: Understanding motivation in chronic illness. *Journal of Occupational Therapy, 48,* 311–317.

Hemphill, B.J. (1988). *Mental health assessment in occupational therapy.* New York: McGraw Hill.

Kemp, B. (1990). Motivational dynamic in geriatric rehabilitation: Toward a therapeutic model. In B. Kemp, K. Brummell-Smith, & J. Ramsdell (Eds.), *Geriatric rehabilitation.* Boston: College-Hill Press.

Kramer, J.J., & Conoley, J.C. (Eds.). (1992). *The eleventh mental measures yearbook.* Lincoln: University of Nebraska Press.

Miller, W., & Rollnick, S. (1991). *Motivational interviewing: Preparing people to change addictive behavior.* New York: Guilford Press.

Mosqueda, L. (1993). Assessment of rehabilitation potential. *Geriatric Rehabilitation, 9,* 689–700.

Neistadt, M. (1995). Methods of assessing clients' priorities: A survey of adult physical dysfunction settings. *American Journal of Occupational Therapy, 49,* 428–436.

Prochaska, J.O., & DiClemente, C.C. (1986). Transtheoretical therapy: Toward a more integrative model of change. *Psychotherapy: Research, Theory and Practice, 19,* 276–288.

Ramsden, E. (1988). Compliance and motivation. *Topics in Geriatric Rehabilitation, 3*(3), 1–14.

Rosenfeld, M.S. (1994). *Measure of subacute rehabilitation potential.* Unpublished.

Schunk, C. (1988). Prediction and assessment of compliant behavior. *Topics in Geriatric Rehabilitation, 3*(3), 15–20.

Thibodaux, L., & Shewchuk, R. (1988). Strategies for compliance in the elderly. *Topics in Geriatric Rehabilitation, 3*(3), 21–33.

Van Etten (1995). Unpublished pilot study. Worchester, MA: Worchester State College.

Versluys, H.P. (1995). Evaluation of emotional adjustment to disabilities. In C. Trombly (Ed.), *Occupational therapy for physical dysfunction* (4th ed., pp. 225–234). Baltimore: Williams & Wilkins.

Index

Contractual agreements between managed care organizations and providers, 153–154

Control
case studies, 63–66, 81–83, 109–110
and group programs, 141

Cooking groups, 142. *See also* Functional retraining groups

Copayments
determination of amounts, 150
and Medicare, 150, 151, 153

Cost issues. *See* Financial issues

Crisis theory, 31–32

Cultural context. *See also* Faith and religion
case study, 81–83
and group programs, 138–139
and home health occupational therapy, 122, 123–124
values, perceptions, and attitudes about money and finances, 154–156

D

Data gathering. *See* Assessments; Evaluations

Declarative memory, 46, 51

Deductibles, 150

Delivery of services
institutional constraints on, 153–154
preserving services through documentation, 97–98

Dementia, 26

Dependency, case studies, 56–59, 61–63, 66–69, 78–80, 179–184

Depression
and ambivalence about aging and health care in America, 11
and assessment, 176
case studies, 60–61, 66–69, 110–111
in developmentally disabled adults, 116
and geropsychiatry, 109
theory and practice in evaluation and treatment, 29, 30, 34–35

The Depression, 155

Development of groups, 130–133, 142

Developmental challenges of aging, 10–11

Developmentally disabled adults
case studies, 61–63, 116
challenges presented by, 115
needs of, 115–118

Dieticians, 125

Disability. *See* Illness and injury; *specific type of disability by name*

Discharge planning
case studies, 59–60, 66–69, 71–74, 109–110, 110–111, 142–145
and group programs, 129–130

Disengagement, case study, 66–69

Doctors, and contractual agreements, 153–154

Documentation
and ambivalence about aging and health care in America, 18
case studies, 95–96, 97
challenges of
effectiveness, 99–101
efficiency, 100, 101
quality, 100, 101
value, 100, 101
forms of, 103–104
in group programs, 132, 133
identifying good writing, 98–99
importance of, 93–94
items to include in, 105
preserving services through, 97–98
and reimbursement of motivational interventions, 93–103
therapists' attitudes about, 96–97
tips for, 102–103
the writing process, 94–96

Dorfzaun, Rhoda, 85–87

Drawing With the Right Side of Your Brain, 103

Drawings in documentation, 102, 103–104

Durable medical equipment, 151, 152. *See also* Assistive equipment

Dying patients, case study, 76–78

E

Eating. *See also* Nutritional services
safe eating, 117–118

Education groups, 131, 142

Edwards, Betty, 103

Effectiveness, as challenge of documentation, 99–101

Efficiency, as challenge of documentation, 100, 101

The Eleventh Mental Measures Yearbook, 173–174

Emotional factors. *See* Psychosocial factors

Empowerment of clients, 33–34